Essentials of Health Care Organization Finance

Essentials of Health Care Organization Finance

A Primer for Board Members

DENNIS D. POINTER
DENNIS M. STILLMAN

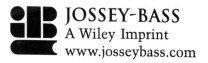

JOSSEY-BASS
A Wiley Imprint
www.josseybass.com

Published by Jossey-Bass
A Wiley Imprint
989 Market Street, San Francisco, CA 94103-1741   www.josseybass.com

Jossey-Bass books and products are available through most bookstores. To contact Jossey-Bass directly call our Customer Care Department within the U.S. at (800) 956-7739, outside the U.S. at (317) 572-3986 or fax (317) 572-4002.

Jossey-Bass also publishes its books in a variety of electronic formats. Some content that appears in print may not be available in electronic books.

Library of Congress Cataloging-in-Publication Data

Pointer, Dennis Dale.
   Essentials of health care organization finance: a primer for board members/ Dennis D. Pointer, Dennis M. Stillman.—1st ed.
       p.; cm.
   Includes index.
   ISBN 0-7879-7403-X (alk. paper)
   1. Health facilities—Finance. 2. Health facilities—Business management. 3. Hospital trustees.
   [DNLM: 1. Financial Management—methods. 2. Health Facilities—economics. 3. Governing Board—standards. WX 157 P752h 2004]
I. Stillman, Dennis M., 1949– II. Title.
   RA971.3.P656 2004
   362.1'068'1—dc22

                                                    2004014543

Printed in the United States of America
FIRST EDITION
HB Printing   10 9 8 7 6 5 4 3 2 1

CONTENTS

LIST OF EXHIBITS

FOREWORD

This book needed to be written. It *must* be read by board members who lack grounding in the basics of accounting and finance or those needing a refresher.

Health care organizations face significant financial challenges: enhancing revenues, managing costs, achieving healthy margins, maintaining creditworthiness, accessing capital at reasonable rates, and ensuring the integrity of financial reporting. Simultaneously, boards are being held to much higher standards of financial responsibility and accountability. Gone are the days when a few financially savvy directors can or should carry a board composed of members who didn't understand "the money aspects" of providing health care.

This book covers all the essentials: foundational accounting concepts, reading and analyzing financial statements, financial planning and budgeting, sources of financing and creditworthiness, capital allocation, and the audit. The treatment is governance-focused and director-friendly. After reading *Essentials of Health Care Organization Finance,* directors will understand a health care organization's financial "anatomy" and "physiology," appreciate their board's financial responsibilities and be better prepared to fulfill them, and have a solid foundation for learning more through their experience of governing.

Every issue on a board's agenda—whether strategic, operation, or clinical—has financial implications and consequences. In order to deal with them effectively and creatively, all directors must possess basic financial literacy. This book lifts the financial fog that many directors experience in their boardrooms.

R. Timothy Stack
President and CEO
Piedmont Medical Center
Atlanta, Georgia

Gregory Hurst
Executive Vice President
and Chief Financial Officer
Piedmont Medical Center
Atlanta, Georgia

Charles W. Wickliffe, M.D.
Board Chair
Piedmont Medical Center
Atlanta, Georgia

PREFACE

This is a book for health care organization board members not formally trained in accounting and finance, which is most of us. We know that understanding the money is important to fulfilling our role as a director. But realizing the need to develop basic financial literacy, and then beginning to do something about it, brings on symptoms like a bad case of the flu. The reason: it is an area riddled with jargon, formulas, technicalities, and column after column after column of numbers (typically in very small print); it's arcane, seemingly complex, and a bit overwhelming. Our best intentions to grasp this stuff wane. Fret no more; this book will help—we guarantee it!

PREMISES

First, the quality of governance matters. It has a significant impact on the performance of health care organizations, the people they serve, and their medical staffs and employees. As a director, you assume an awesome responsibility: stewardship of your community's most precious resource. Second, health care organizations are businesses and must be financially sound to remain in business. One of your most important roles as a director is to ensure this. Third, all issues coming before your board—strategic, operational, and clinical—have financial implications. Fourth, to govern wisely, effectively, and creatively, you must understand and be able to employ basic accounting and finance concepts. Fifth, your board must receive useful, meaningful, accurate, and timely financial information. The focus, form, and format of this information are quite different from what is required by financial professionals and executives.

APPROACH

The book has some unique features, making it unlike most accounting or finance texts you'll encounter. It is *tightly crafted*. All unnecessary detail has been eliminated; this will be a quick and efficient read. *The approach is non-technical*. The dense fog that usually hangs over this area is lifted; accounting and finance, at the level directors must understand it, is not complicated. *Only the most important basics are included*—those things you must understand to fulfill your director responsibilities. We *assume that you have no previous knowledge* of accounting or finance and its application to health care organizations. This book is totally self-contained; it builds every key idea from the ground up. The book *focuses on the financial activities* in which your board is engaged, the issues it faces, and information it needs to govern. Each chapter *is loaded with illustrations and recommendations* that help you begin using what you're learning in the boardroom.

ORGANIZATION

Every chapter addresses a critical area or issue that you must understand to fulfill the financial aspect of your director role. The chapters build on one another, so we recommend reading them in order.

Here's a roadmap of the journey ahead:

Chapter One: Governing

Your board's obligations, responsibilities, and roles—the *why, what,* and *how* aspects of governing

The nature of governance work

Factors that most affect your board's performance and contributions

Ratio analysis of financial statements: liquidity, profitability, capital structure, activity, and operating

Board financial oversight

Chapter Seven: Looking Forward—Vision, Strategies, Financial Plans, and Budgets

The planning cycle: visioning and strategic planning

Financial planning and plans

Budgeting and budgets

Board oversight of financial plans

Chapter Eight: Source of Funds—Financing

Capital structure: your organization's mix of equity and debt financing

Creditworthiness and factors affecting it

Bonds and bond ratings

Securing long-term debt

Chapter Nine: Use of Funds—Capital Investment

The capital cycle

Types of capital projects

Your board's role in the capital investment process

Approaches to capital decision making

Payback analysis

Net present value analysis

Nonfinancial criteria used to assess capital projects

Chapter Ten: Financial Integrity and Credibility

Ensuring financial soundness and legitimacy: your board's role

Subdivision of functions and tasks: your board and its audit committee

The audit

Internal controls

Your board's financial responsibility and accountability: changing expectations and standards

Chapter Eleven: The Finale

Big blips that should be on your board's financial radar screen

Checklist: assessing your board's financial fitness and savvy

Resources for learning more

Each chapter (with the exception of Three, Four, and Eleven) concludes with a section called "In the Boardroom"—our recommendations for beginning to apply what you're learning to the practice of governing.

Dennis Pointer conducts about twenty board retreats a year for health care organizations and gives an equal number of speeches on various governance topics to national, state, and local trade and professional associations. At these events, someone always asks, "What can I do to increase my financial IQ?" Until now, he didn't have a good recommendation. Even though there are a number of books on accounting and finance for health administration students and executives, nothing is available that meets the needs of board members. He now has an answer. This book needed to be written.

This was a team effort by a pair of colleagues whose offices at the University of Washington are less than fifty feet apart: a "governance guy" who knows some accounting and finance and an "accounting/finance guy" who really understands governance. We've learned a lot from each other in planning and writing this book, and we hope that you'll benefit from the synergy. If you want to give us feedback or have a comment, please contact us.

ACKNOWLEDGMENTS

Andrew Pasternack, senior editor at Jossey-Bass, has been the go-to guy for Dennis Pointer's last three books in addition to this one. He's a valued friend (always buffering the inherent tension between publisher and author), wise counselor, gentle but firm prodder to meet all those deadlines, and Magellanlike navigator of lengthy and complex journeys. We thank our colleagues who reviewed the book for clarity of presentation and technical accuracy: Jan Jennings, president and CEO of American Healthcare Solutions, LLC (and former CEO of Jefferson Regional Medical Center in Pittsburgh; Children's Memorial Medical Center in Chicago; and Millard Fillmore Hospitals in Buffalo, New York); Craig Goodrich, CPA, vice president and chief financial officer of Virginia Mason Medical Center (Seattle, Washington); Leann Dawson, CPA, controller of the University of Washington Medical Center (Seattle); and Maureen Broom, CPA, Department of Accounting, University of Washington Medical Center (Seattle). The standard disclaimer really does apply here: Andy, Jan, Craig, Leann, and Maureen did their best, but we bear responsibility for all the flaws.

Yes, accounting and finance can be fun and interesting; we hope you enjoy, and benefit from, this book. We tip our hats to *you*, volunteer directors who freely contribute your knowledge, skills, wisdom, and time to making the U.S. health system the world's best.

Dennis D. Pointer
Austin Ross Professor of Health Care
  Management
Department of Health Services
School of Public Health and
  Community Medicine
University of Washington, Seattle
dpointer@u.washington.edu

President
Dennis D. Pointer & Associates
Seattle, Washington
(206) 632–6066
dennis.pointer@comcast.net

Dennis M. Stillman
Associate Director and Senior Lecturer
Program in Health Services
  Administration
School of Public Health and
  Community Medicine
University of Washington
(206) 221–7234
stillman@u.washington.edu

Dennis M. Stillman Associates
Seattle, Washington
(206) 459-1846
stillmanassoc@w-link.net

ABOUT THE AUTHORS

Dennis D. Pointer is one of the nation's foremost governance consultants, advisors, speakers, and writers. He is the author of more than seventy articles and eight books, among them *Really Governing, Board Work, Getting to Great: Principles of Health Care Organization Governance, The High Performance Board,* and *The Health Care Industry: A Primer for Board Members. Really Governing* and *Board Work* have won the James A. Hamilton Book of the Year Award from the American College of Healthcare Executives. Pointer has been the chair or a member of more than twenty boards.

His firm, Dennis D. Pointer & Associates, provides governance consulting, retreat facilitation, assessment, and design and development services. DDP&A has worked with more than 450 health systems and hospitals, nonprofit organizations, commercial corporations, and government agencies to improve their governance performance and contributions. He is also vice president and partner of the American Governance and Leadership Group, LLC; sponsored by the American Hospital, it provides board education and development services to health care organizations.

Pointer is Austin Ross Professor, Department of Health Services, University of Washington School of Public Health and Community Medicine. He has held two previous endowed chairs: the John J. Hanlon Professorship of Health Services Research and Policy, Graduate School of Public Health, San Diego State University (1991–2002 and currently *emeritus*); and the Arthur Graham Glasgow Chair of Health Services Management at the Medical College of Virginia (1986–1991). From 1975 to 1986 he was affiliated with the University of California, Los Angeles, where he served as professor and chairman, Department of Health Services Management, School of Public Health; and associate director, UCLA Medical Center. During his tenure at UCLA, he was a senior fellow at the RAND Corporation. He has held faculty appointments at the University of Iowa, Mount Sinai School of Medicine, and the Baruch School of Management of the City University of New York.

Pointer is a recipient of the Foster G. McGaw Medal of Excellence in Health Administration, Education, and Research. He received his B.Sc. degree in organizational psychology from Iowa State University and Ph.D. in health administration from the University of Iowa.

Dennis M. Stillman is senior lecturer and associate director, Program in Health Services Administration, University of Washington School of Public Health and Community Medicine, where he teaches graduate-level courses in accounting and finance. He is an adjunct faculty member at San Diego State University (Graduate School of Public Health) and Seattle Pacific University. His firm, Dennis M. Stillman Associates, provides financial consulting, interim chief financial officer services, financial leadership coaching, and financial education for trustees, physician leaders, and health care managers.

Before making the transition to academia, Stillman was, for twelve years, associate administrator and chief financial officer of the University of Washington Medical Center (UWMC). During his tenure at UWMC, it was consistently ranked among the top hospitals in the country by *U.S. News and World Report*. He has held previous positions as vice president and chief financial officer, Pacific Medical Center (Seattle, Washington); controller, Marshall Hale Memorial Hospital (San Francisco); assistant administrator, Sonoma Valley Hospital District (California); auditor, Arthur Andersen; and chief accountant, Valley Medical Center (Renton, Washington).

Stillman received his B.A. in business administration from the University of Puget Sound and M.H.A. from the University of Washington. He is a certified public accountant–inactive and fellow of the Healthcare Financial Management Association.

Essentials of
Health Care
Organization
Finance

CHAPTER 1

Governing

OBJECTIVES

After completing this chapter, you will understand:

- Your board's obligation to stakeholders
- The nature of governance work (responsibilities and roles)
- Factors that most affect your board's performance and contributions

---

gov•ern [gûv' `ern], verb; syn. guide, direct, control
Exercise ultimate authority and accountability
Represent the interests of an organization's owners
    as an agent or trustee
What boards do

Health system boards, hospital boards, medical group boards, home health agency boards, health plan boards, health maintenance organization (HMO) boards, professional association boards . . . there are approximately thirty thousand boards in the health care industry, and about 330,000 people serve on them. They govern nonprofit organizations, commercial corporations, and government agencies ranging from small, local institutions to multibillion dollar enterprises national in scope.

Health care organization boards are a diverse lot. But beyond some superficial differences, they are identical in terms of their obligations, responsibilities, and roles (see Exhibit 1.1).

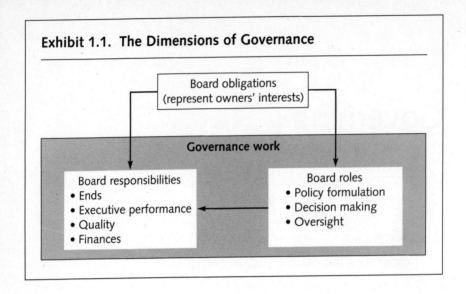

Exhibit 1.1. The Dimensions of Governance

Board obligations
(represent owners' interests)

Governance work

Board responsibilities
- Ends
- Executive performance
- Quality
- Finances

Board roles
- Policy formulation
- Decision making
- Oversight

OBLIGATIONS

Every board exists to represent the interest of an organization's owners: stockholders in commercial corporations, stakeholders in nonprofits, constituents in government agencies. The overarching obligation of a board is to ensure an organization's resources and capacities are deployed in ways that benefit its owners.

Organizations are collections of resources: money, people, facilities, equipment, supplies, capabilities. They are *means*. Their *end* is benefiting those who own them. Boards make sure this is the case; this is the *why* aspect of governance. For nonprofit health care organization boards, the essence of the verb "governing" is advancing and protecting the interests of stakeholders, serving as their agent, and deciding and acting on their behalf.

The owners of commercial corporations are easily identified (everyone who owns stock); additionally, they have roughly similar objectives (wealth enhancement). Things are not so simple in nonprofits. Stakeholders are often vaguely defined (such as "the community") and they typically want different things, some of which can be in conflict with one another. To represent stakeholders, boards must specifically identify the key ones and then understand their needs, demands, and expectations. Governing begins here.

The Board's Fiduciary Duty of Loyalty

All state incorporation laws require boards and directors to discharge a fiduciary duty of loyalty. Loyalty holds that directors, in performing their roles, owe allegiance to the organization and its stakeholders, acting in their best interest rather than for personal gain or the benefit of other organizations, groups, and individuals. All dealings, actions, and decisions of directors in their official capacity must meet two requirements. First, they must have *good faith* intentions, manifesting honesty and a genuine desire to discharge their obligation. Second, they must behave in ways that demonstrate *reasonable belief* their decisions and actions are in the best interest of the organization and its stakeholders.

Health care organization directors breach their duty of loyalty when, for example, a material conflict of interest influences a decision; they disclose confidential information that could have a detrimental effect on the organization; they seize a business opportunity for themselves or other parties that legitimately belongs to the organization; or, in nonprofit, they vote for an unlawful distribution of the organization's assets that subverts its charitable purpose or results in private inurement.

RESPONSIBILITIES

Peter Drucker succinctly defines effectiveness as "doing the right things." To govern effectively, a health care organization board must fulfill four responsibilities and sets of associated duties; this is the *what* aspect of governance.

Responsibility	Duties
Organizational ends	• Formulating a vision; a precise, explicit, "fine-grained," and empowering notion of what the organization should become (on behalf of stakeholders) at its very best, in the future

Organizational ends *(continued)*	• Specifying key goals; the organization's most important specific "accomplishables"; what must be achieved to fulfill the vision
	• Making sure management strategies are aligned with (and lead to achieving) key goals and the vision
Executive performance	• Selecting the chief executive officer (CEO)
	• Specifying expectations of the CEO
	• Assessing the CEO's performance and contributions
	• Adjusting the CEO's compensation
	• Terminating the CEO's employment, should the need arise
Quality of care	• Appointing, reappointing, and determining privileges of medical staff members
	• Ensuring that necessary quality, utilization, and risk management systems are in place and functioning effectively
	• Monitoring and assessing the quality of care provided and, if problems are detected, expecting corrective action
Organizational financial health	• This responsibility is the focus of Chapter Two

A board must fulfill these four responsibilities, which are legally mandated and functionally necessary. There are many other things that a board and its directors can, and might choose, to do: make personal contributions or solicit funds for the organization, serve as an organizational advocate and spokesperson, and offer advice and counsel to the CEO. Though adding great value if done well, they are optional. Suggestions for performing these tasks are given in the sidebar "Other Board Tasks."

Other Board Tasks

Directors have the right, and may be encouraged, to make personal financial contributions to the organization. However, such contributions should never be the only (or even an important) prerequisite for being nominated to, or continuing to serve on, the board.

Directors often have access to potential donors. Because of their commitment to, investment in, and knowledge of the organization, they can be very helpful soliciting contributions. However, fundraising should be viewed as a supplemental (even a peripheral) activity of the board; it should never overwhelm, displace, or jeopardize fulfilling core governing responsibilities. Fundraising is a distinctive organizational function that is often most effectively conducted by a separate foundation with its own board.

Serving as an advocate for the organization is something expected of every director. However, they should be careful speaking on behalf of the organization; too many people doing so in an uncoordinated way can send confusing and conflicting messages that could do more harm than good. When it is necessary for someone to talk with key external constituents about important issues, consider having the board chair, accompanied by the CEO, make the presentation.

CEOs often, and appropriately, seek counsel from the board chair and individual directors on substantive issues related to the performance of their managerial roles. Because of their familiarity with the organization (in addition to standing outside of it), directors can be quite helpful. But the key here is that when offering such counsel, a director is not acting in a governance capacity and the advice can be accepted or rejected.

ROLES

To fulfill its responsibilities, a board must perform three roles: formulating policies, making decisions, and engaging in oversight. These are the *how* aspects of governance.

Formulating Policies

It is by formulating policies that a board influences an organization, ensuring that it benefits stakeholders and advances their interests. Board policies are declarative statements that direct and constrain subsequent decisions and actions. They are mechanisms for performing two absolutely essential governance functions: first, expressing board expectations of management and the medical staff, conveying what it wants done (acceptable methods) and accomplished (desired results); and second, setting policies that specify delegated authorities and tasks.

Decision Making

Ask what the most important thing a board does, and the answer is typically to make decisions. But board decisions must be grounded on, and flow from, policies (absent this, they risk being idiosyncratic and disjointed) and deal only with the most important organizational issues requiring governance-level involvement. A board has four decision-making options:

1. Retain authority and make a decision itself

2. Request proposals and recommendations (from management and the medical staff) and then decide

3. Delegate decision-making authority with constraints; a decision is handed off to management or the medical staff, but with limitations

4. Delegate decision making by exception; management and the medical staff are authorized to make all decisions in a given area, with the exception of those that have been expressly prohibited or reserved by the board

Essentials of Health Care Organization Finance

Examples of Decisions Boards Make

- Are the strategies proposed by management appropriately aligned with key organizational goals and the vision? Should they be approved? (This is a decision regarding *ends*.)
- Did the CEO meet board-specified performance objectives last year? How much of a bonus should he or she be awarded? (This is a decision regarding *executive performance*.)
- Should Dr. _____ be reappointed to the medical staff? Which diseases should she be allowed to treat, and which procedures should she be authorized to perform? (This is a decision regarding *quality*.)
- Should a new audit firm be retained? (This is a decision regarding *finances*.)

Board Policy

There are four different types of policies (see Exhibit 1.2). The board can convey its expectations and directives by being prescriptive (stating "thou shalts") or by being prohibitive (stating "thou shalt nots"). Additionally, policies can focus on either methods or results.

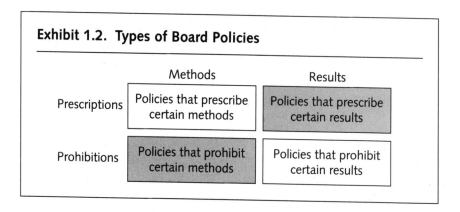

Exhibit 1.2. Types of Board Policies

	Methods	Results
Prescriptions	Policies that prescribe certain methods	Policies that prescribe certain results
Prohibitions	Policies that prohibit certain methods	Policies that prohibit certain results

The most effective policies *prescribe results* and *prohibit methods*. Results are what a board wants accomplished. The best way of conveying them is simply saying "achieve this." As a general rule, a board should avoid specifying methods; there are an infinite number of them, and getting involved in determining the way results are to be achieved bogs a board down in detail. Also, prescribing one method eliminates all others. Doing so takes a board dangerously near, if not across, the line that separates governing from managing. Therefore, if a board must express expectations regarding methods, we recommend formulating policies that restrict, limit, and prohibit—clearly denoting those that are unacceptable.

Engaging in Oversight

The dashboard of your car doesn't give a lot of information. But try driving without it—no gas gauge, speedometer, odometer, battery indicator, oil pressure light, or engine thermometer. In performing the oversight role, a board monitors and assesses key organizational processes and outcomes, answering four questions:

1. Is the organization performing in a manner that protects and advances stakeholder interests?

2. Are the board's expectations, as conveyed in its policies, being met?

3. Are board decisions having the desired impact?

4. Are board directives and constraints being respected as management and the medical staff perform delegated tasks?

GOVERNANCE WORK

A board's job is to formulate policies; make decisions; and oversee ends, executive performance, quality, and finances.

As depicted in Exhibit 1.3, governance work is a three-by-four matrix. To govern effectively, a health care organization board must fill all twelve cells.

The work of a board, when contrasted with the work of management and clinicians, is distinctive for several reasons. First, governance is the ul-

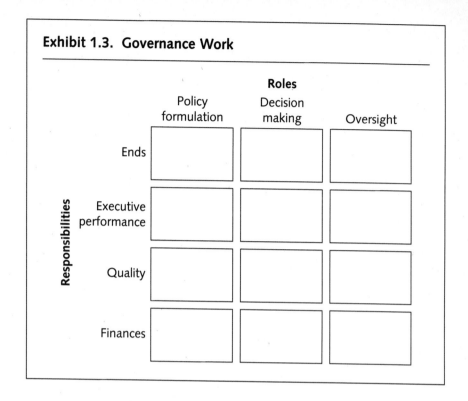

Exhibit 1.3. Governance Work

	Roles		
Responsibilities	Policy formulation	Decision making	Oversight
Ends			
Executive performance			
Quality			
Finances			

timate team sport. A board decides and acts only as a group. Individual directors have no authority or power. Second, it is part-time work. Other key leadership groups have a continuous presence in the organization, but boards do not; they come and go. Third, governance work is fragmented. A board convenes, does its work, and then adjourns. Weeks or months pass before the directors meet again. As a consequence, thrust, follow-through, and follow-up can be difficult to sustain.

GOVERNANCE "ENABLERS"

The work of governing is influenced by a board's structure, composition, and infrastructure.

Structure is the way governance work is subdivided and coordinated, including: board size; number and type of board committees; and, in a system, the number of governing layers and boards. *Composition* is the characteristics of directors in addition to their knowledge, skills, and experience. *Infrastructure* comprises resources such as budget, staff, and information systems.

IN THE BOARDROOM

➤ Get a copy of your board's bylaws and review them.

➤ Ask for a briefing on your organization's directors and officers (D and O) indemnification policy and liability insurance coverage. It's prudent to have your personal attorney review these documents. In making this suggestion, the intent is not to scare you. Health care organization boards and directors are rarely successfully sued. But keep in mind that there are potential liabilities associated with board service.

➤ If you have not had an orientation to the organization (its facilities, programs and services, management team, market and competitors), ask for one.

➤ Review your organization's vision and mission statement(s) and key goals.

➤ Has your board done a stakeholder analysis? That is, have you mapped key organizational stakeholders and their most important needs and expectations? It's impossible for your board to effectively represent the interest of stakeholders if it hasn't identified them.

➤ Does your board have a precise, coherent, and shared fix on its obligation, responsibilities, and roles? Your board will not be effective if directors have differing definitions of the why, what, and how aspects of governance.

CHAPTER 2

Financial Responsibilities

OBJECTIVES

After completing this chapter, you will understand:

- Some of the financial challenges facing health care organizations
- The nature and scope of your board's financial responsibilities
- The type of work your board's finance committee should be doing

Health care organization financial challenges are far greater than (and of a very different type from) those faced in the past. Here are a few illustrations:

- Expenditures for health care have increased from 5 percent of gross domestic product in 1960 to approximately 15 percent ($1.6 trillion) in 2003. This rate of growth is unsustainable. As a consequence, health care organizations will experience mounting demands (from Medicare, Medicaid, health plans, and corporate purchasers of health services) to control their costs.
- Competition has increased significantly in most local health care markets. For example, hospitals compete not only with each other but also with their own medical staffs and an array of other providers, including outpatient surgery and urgent care centers, specialty hospitals that focus only on specific diseases, and freestanding diagnostic facilities.

- Health care organization revenues have come under increased pressure from federal reimbursement restrictions, capitation, and aggressive contract negotiations by insurance companies, health plans, and HMOs.
- Health care organizations face increasing demands on their limited resources to improve the quality of patient care and safety, modernize facilities, install state-of-the-art information systems, expand services and programs, acquire the next generation of clinical technologies, and keep wages of highly trained personnel competitive.
- Many health care organizations have become huge, diverse, and complex business enterprises, often with revenues in the billions of dollars.

During the 1960s, 1970s, and 1980s, the survival of health care organizations was pretty much assured; few experienced severe financial difficulties and bankruptcies were rare. By the 1990s, and into the early years of this century, their viability is no longer guaranteed.

At the same time, boards are being subjected to heightened financial expectations and standards. In large measure, this is the result of well-publicized organization debacles, such as the Allegheny Health Education and Research Foundation (AHERF), PhyCor, HealthSouth—due, in part, to problematic board oversight. Bond rating agencies and insurers, institutional lenders, accrediting organizations, foundations, major donors, the press, and the public are demanding far greater financial accountability and transparency.

As noted in Chapter One, a board has four core responsibilities, one of which is ensuring the organization's financial health. To fulfill this responsibility, it must:

- Formulate the organization's financial objectives
- Ensure that management's plans and budgets are aligned with, and lead to accomplishing, board-specified financial objectives
- Monitor or assess financial performance and outcomes, and require development of corrective measures if deficiencies are detected
- Make sure that necessary internal controls are in place, oversee the audit, and ensure that financial statements fairly reflect the organization's condition

Essentials of Health Care Organization Finance

The relationship of these four duties and their linkage with an organization's vision and key goals are portrayed in Exhibit 2.1. Financial objectives must be grounded on, and flow from, a board-formulated vision and management's strategic plans. This forms the foundation for board oversight of financial plans, financial performance, and financial controls.

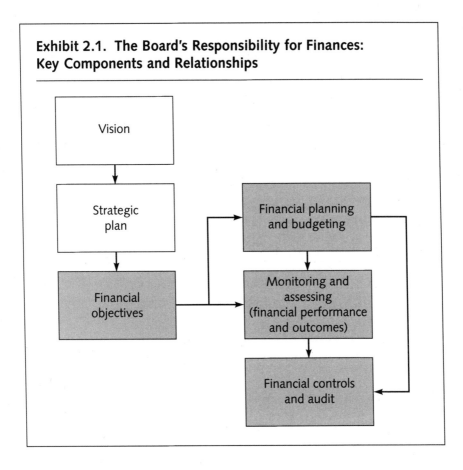

Exhibit 2.1. The Board's Responsibility for Finances: Key Components and Relationships

OBJECTIVES

The board's responsibility begins with formulating and updating annual financial objectives for the organization. The objectives should answer three questions: What is the board's definition of financial health? What must the organization achieve financially to fulfill its vision? How should the organization's financial performance and condition be assessed?

Objectives can focus on ends or means. Ends-oriented objectives specify desired results; means-oriented objectives denote actions a board wants undertaken.

Board-level financial objectives should:

- Focus on the long run
- Deal with only those things that are most vision-critical
- Be few in number, typically no more than fifteen
- Be clearly stated
- Be unequivocal (words such as *may* and *should* must be avoided)
- Contain a precise target (quantitatively stated, where possible) and date by which it is to be achieved

The process of formulating financial objectives must be boardcentric. Although management and physician leaders need to be consulted and weigh in, such objectives must be an expression of the board's expectations and a product of its deliberation.

Illustrative Board-Formulated Financial Objectives

- Each year the organization will achieve a net profit margin of at least ___ percent.
- Operating revenues will grow at an annual rate of ___ percent over the next ___ years.
- The organization will maintain an "A" bond rating.
- Severity-adjusted cost per inpatient discharge will be reduced ___ percent by the first quarter of 200__.
- Net yield on investment income (adjusted for inflation, less transaction costs and management fees) will be at least ___ percent per year.

PLANS

Financial plans and budgets (the subject of Chapter Seven) are management tools and the means for allocating an organization's resources to achieve financial objectives.

Overwhelmed by the detail and complexity in addition to the amount of time and effort invested in preparation of plans and budgets, a board's involvement here is often far more symbolic than substantive. The board must approve financial plans and review budgets. However, the type of financial information that management requires to run the organization is not the same as what the board needs to govern it. Management should prepare governance-friendly plans and budgets composed of summary categories, rather than specific line items. An accompanying rationale should describe how each category leads to achieving, and is aligned with, board-specified financial objectives and the vision.

In reviewing financial plans and budgets, the board must probe and question, asking:

- What are the assumptions on which the plan's success depends?
- How aggressive is the plan? To what extent does it stretch the organization's capacities and competencies?
- What could go wrong? What execution problems could be expected?
- What financial targets must be achieved, and how will they be monitored and evaluated?

MONITORING AND ASSESSING

Board-specified financial objectives and approved plans and budgets are the basis for monitoring and assessing the organization's financial performance and outcomes. Four steps are required:

1. *Developing key indicators.* They are based on financial objectives (an example of a measure might be net income from operations), variations in budget projections from actual results, and ratios calculated from the organization's financial statements.

2. *Specifying standards.* For example, if the objective is to achieve a net income from operations of 4 percent, the target percentage becomes the standard.

3. *Assessing.* Compare actual performance to the standard.

4. *Controlling.* If deficiencies are detected, expect management to develop and undertake corrective action.

CONTROLS AND THE AUDIT

Boards are ultimately accountable for ensuring that accounting systems for supplying accurate, reliable, and timely information are in place and functioning effectively; transactions are properly authorized, executed, and recorded; funds are expended for legitimate purposes in appropriate ways; and financial statements fairly reflect the organization's financial condition.

This is often accomplished through an annual audit performed for the board by a public accounting firm. It examines the organization's books and financial statements, ascertains whether procedures and practices conform to generally accepted accounting principles (GAAP), and transmits opinions and recommendations. Some organizations do not have annual audits. In these instances, an internal audit function—even without an internal auditor—is critical. Financial controls and the audit are the focus of Chapter Ten.

ORGANIZATION

In discharging its responsibility for finances, a board should be assisted by a finance committee. Core functions of this committee should include:

• Reviewing management-developed financial plans and budgets; passing recommendations on to the board for input and approval

• Reviewing all management proposals regarding operational and capital expenditures that exceed board-preapproved authorization limits; sending recommendations to the board for review, input, and action

- Annually forwarding a memo to the board assessing the organization's overall financial performance and condition
- Drafting policies regarding finances; sending them to the board for review, input, and action
- Reviewing and analyzing proposals submitted by management regarding finances; sending them to the board for review, input, and action
- Drafting decisions regarding finances that must be made by the board; sending them to the board for review, input, and action
- Recommending quantitative measures to be employed by the board for assessing the organization's financial performance
- Directing and overseeing the investment of funds:

> Selecting investment advisors
>
> Developing investment objectives and criteria
>
> Assessing investment advisors and fund performance
>
> Making recommendations to the executive committee and board for their review, input, and action

- Undertaking an annual assessment of all board policies and decisions regarding finances

The finance committee should be chaired by a director who is knowledgeable and experienced in the area of accounting and finance. Members should possess basic financial literacy or be expected to develop it. The CEO and CFO should either sit on the committee *ex officio* with a vote or attend all meetings.

IN THE BOARDROOM

➤ Request that management give your board periodic briefings regarding the financial climate (and associated opportunities and threats) of the health care industry.

➤ Do directors have a precise, explicit, and shared notion of your board's financial responsibilities and duties? If not, your board may want to consider devoting a portion of a board retreat to discussing them and how they should be discharged.

➤ Does your board have a finance committee? Does it perform the functions denoted in the previous section?

➤ What is your board's level of financial literacy? Do directors possess the basic knowledge necessary to fulfill your board's responsibility for ensuring the organization's financial health and continuing viability? This is critical because it gives directors confidence to ask questions, understand the answers, and press when things are not clear.

CHAPTER 3

Health Care Industry Financial Structure and Dynamics

OBJECTIVES

After completing this chapter, you will understand:

- The nature, magnitude, and scope of the U.S. health care industry
- The flow of funds through the system—where the money comes from and how it's spent
- The nature of health insurance and health plans

A Note on This Chapter

This chapter is based on material previously published in *The Health Care Industry: A Primer for Board Members,* by Dennis Pointer and Stephen Williams (Jossey-Bass, 2003).

We have chosen not to pepper these pages with citations though we have drawn on a number of sources. Unless otherwise noted, all data are taken from government sources in the public domain:

Chartbook on Trends in the Health of Americans (Hyattsville, Md.: National Center for Health Statistics, 2002)

(*Continued*)

Health, United States—2002 (Hyattsville, Md.: National Center for Health Statistics, 2002)

Statistical Abstract of the United States, 2001 (Washington, D.C.: U.S. Bureau of the Census, 2001)

Data on health insurance, health plans, and their coverage were drawn from:

Source Book of Health Insurance Data (Washington, D.C.: Health Insurance Institute of America, 2000)

Health Insurance Coverage (Washington, D.C.: Bureau of the Census, 2000)

Health Insurance Coverage and the Uninsured (Washington, D.C.: Health Insurance Institute of America, 1999)

THE BIG PICTURE

In 2002, total health care industry expenditures were $1.3 trillion, accounting for about 13 percent of the gross domestic product (GDP), as compared with $27 billion and 5 percent of GDP in 1960. The United States spends a greater percentage of its GDP on health care than any other industrialized country. An amazing fact: if U.S. health care were a separate economy, it would rank fourth in the world—behind the United States, Japan, and Germany. An overview of the U.S. health care industry is in Exhibit 3.1.

The money to fuel this huge industry comes from two sources: private (employers, individuals, households) and government (federal, state, and local) sources. The distribution has changed dramatically over time: in 1960, 75 percent of total health care expenditures came from private sources and 25 percent was from the government; in 2000 it was 55 percent private funds and 45 percent from government.

The $1.3 trillion spent on health care services and supplies is distributed as shown in Exhibit 3.2. Fully 80 percent is for hospitals, professional services (physicians, dentists, podiatrists, optometrists, and so forth), and retail health products (primarily pharmaceuticals). The largest components, hospital and professional services, are evenly split, about one-third of the total each.

Exhibit 3.1. The U.S. Health Care Industry at a Glance

National Health Care Expenditures

Per year	$1.3 trillion
Per day	$3.6 billion
Per hour	$148 million
Per minute	$2.5 million
Per second	$36,500
Annually per person	$4,000
Percentage of gross domestic product	13%
Percentage from government funds	43%
Percentage from private funds	57%
Percentage spent on provision of personal health care services	87%
Spent on prescription drugs	$122 billion

Health Insurance

With no coverage: number of individuals	41 million
With no coverage: percentage of the population under age 65	17%
Percentage of population that has coverage through:	
Private health insurance (those under age 65)	72%
Private health insurance provided by employer (those under age 65)	67%
Enrollment in a health maintenance organization (those under age 65)	34%
Medicare	14%
Medicaid	9%

General Hospitals

Organizations	5,800
Beds	1 million
Average beds occupied	66%

(*Continued*)

Exhibit 3.1. The U.S. Health Care Industry at a Glance, Cont'd.

Average hospital size	170 beds
Annual inpatient admissions	35 million
Average inpatient stay	6.8 days
Annual (hospital) outpatient visits	85 million
Annual (hospital) emergency room visits	108 million
Annual expenditures	$412 billion
Nursing Homes	
Organizations	17,000
Beds	1.8 million
Average beds occupied	82%
Average daily residents	1.5 million
Annual expenditures	$92 billion
Mental and Behavioral Health	
Psychiatric hospitals	580
Psychiatric units in general hospitals	1,700
Annual expenditures	$33 billion
Personnel	
Total health care industry workforce	12 million
Percentage of all working adults	9%
Physicians	
Number (active)	690,000
Annual office visits	824 million
Annual expenditures	$286 billion
Other Health Care Personnel	
Registered nurses	2.3 million
Pharmacists	208,000
Dentists	168,000
Physical therapists	144,000
Speech therapists	97,000
Podiatrists	11,000

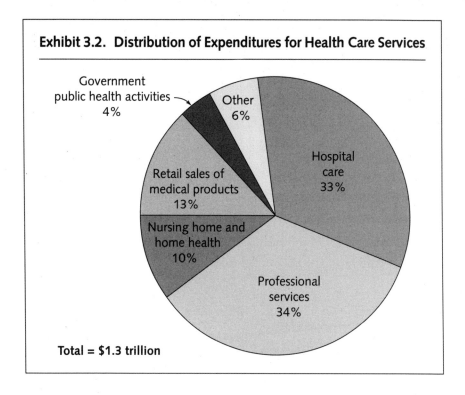

Exhibit 3.2. Distribution of Expenditures for Health Care Services

Government public health activities 4%

Other 6%

Retail sales of medical products 13%

Nursing home and home health 10%

Hospital care 33%

Professional services 34%

Total = $1.3 trillion

In 1960 $23 billion was spent on personal health care services ($126 per person); 1999 expenditures were $1,068 billion ($3,808 per person). Over the past four decades such expenditures have increased in absolute dollars forty-sixfold and per capita thirtyfold, about 10 percent each year.

HEALTH INSURANCE

Health insurance is an umbrella term used to describe a variety of methods for financing provision of health care services.

Insurance spreads the risk of financial loss associated with an event among members of a group. Traditionally, it is provided (underwritten) in those instances where the potential loss (1) is large (catastrophic) and beyond the ability of an individual to pay, (2) has a monetary value, (3) cannot be influenced or controlled by the individual, and (4) is predictable for the group as a whole over a specified period of time. The risks and expenditures associated with the use of most personal health care services do not meet these criteria. For example, routine health care expenditures for an individual or family are small, discretionary, and predictable. Accordingly, health insurance is not technically insurance per se, but rather a form of prepayment where small periodic contributions are made on the basis of the likelihood of future outlays by members of a group. Bowing to convention, the term *health insurance* is used here.

There are three types of health insurance:

1. *Voluntary health insurance,* purchased by employers for their employees or retirees and by individuals from nonprofit and commercial health plans

2. *Social insurance,* provided by a government health plan as a benefit that is earned (such as Medicare)

3. *Public welfare insurance,* provided by government to eligible individuals on the basis of need (for example, Medicaid)

Approximately 84 percent of the population is covered by some form of health insurance, although benefits vary widely. Total enrollment by type of insurance is private 63 percent, Medicare 16 percent, and Medicaid 9 percent (does not exceed 84 percent because of overlapping coverage).

In 2000, forty-one million persons, 17 percent of the population under the age of sixty-five, had no health insurance coverage. The U.S. Census Bureau estimates that those without health insurance will grow to fifty-three to sixty million by 2007, 21–25 percent of the nonelderly population.

VOLUNTARY HEALTH INSURANCE

Voluntary health insurance (VHI) is a diverse array of mechanisms for financing health care services obtained through private (nonprofit and commercial) sources. It is offered by businesses as an employee benefit or purchased directly by individuals. VHI can either serve as the sole source of coverage or supplement benefits offered by social health insurance, such as Medicare (addressed in the next section).

The first VHI plan (making set dollar payments for loss of income due to illness and injury) was offered by Franklin Health Insurance in the 1850s. The number of health insurance companies grew slowly during the late nineteenth and early twentieth centuries. Contemporary VHI can be dated to 1929, when Baylor Hospital in Dallas, Texas, insured a group of public school teachers for in-patient hospital expenses; this was the first Blue Cross plan. Other similar plans were created in the early 1930s. In 1939 the California Medical Society offered VHI to cover in-hospital physician services; this was the first Blue Shield plan.

There are four basic types of VHI:

1. *Commercial* plans can be either nonprofit or for-profit; some are mutuals (owned by their policy holders), others are stock corporations.

2. *Blue Cross and Blue Shield* plans have historical ties to the hospital industry and medical profession, often operate under special state enabling laws, and are generally not subject to the same regulations as commercial plans. Historically, they have been nonprofit entities; in recent years some have converted to for-profit status and many have commercial subsidiaries. These plans are represented nationally by the Blue Cross and Blue Shield Association.

3. *HMOs* (addressed in a subsequent section) combine underwriting (the insurance function) with delivery of health services through an owned or contracted network of providers.

4. *Self-funded* plans are typically sponsored by employers who bear the full financial risk of providing health care benefits to employees, dependents, and retirees. They do not purchase insurance from, or pay premiums to, a health plan; however, they may contract with them to provide administrative services.

Seventy-two percent of the population has some form of VHI; enrollment is roughly split among commercial, Blue Cross plus Blue Shield, and HMO plus self-funded plans. Coverage is generally dependent upon, and linked to, employment. Approximately 50 percent of private sector establishments (employing about 80 percent of the nongovernmental workforce) offer VHI to their employees.

SOCIAL INSURANCE (MEDICARE)

Medicare is the health care industry's single largest payer. In 2000 it covered forty million people (14 percent of the population) and spent $227 billion (about $5,500 per enrollee); $88 billion in Medicare funding went to hospitals, accounting for about 30 percent of their total patient revenues; and $37 billion went to physicians, accounting for about 20 percent of their total revenues.

Medicare was enacted in 1965 as an amendment (Title 18) to the Social Security Act. It is a federally sponsored program that provides health insurance to individuals over sixty-five in addition to disabled persons receiving Social Security benefits and those with end-stage renal disease. Medicare is not welfare; individuals make contributions to the program through payroll deductions and are entitled to receive benefits. The program is managed by the Centers for Medicare and Medicaid Services (CMS).

Medicare is actually two separate, though coordinated, programs: *Part A* is a compulsory health plan that covers hospital-based services; *Part B* is a voluntary, supplemental plan that covers professional (primarily physician) services.

Medicare Part A

Regarding *financing*, Medicare Part A hospital insurance is funded by payroll taxes paid into the Social Security Trust Fund. Employees contribute 1.45 percent of wages, matched equally by employers; self-employed individuals pay 2.9 percent of earnings.

The program provides a number of *benefits*: ninety days of inpatient hospital care per episode of illness; a lifetime reserve of sixty days of inpatient

Essentials of Health Care Organization Finance

hospital care, which can be drawn upon when the maximum for an episode is exceeded; and home health visits following an inpatient admission.

For each episode of illness, beneficiaries make *payments* of a deductible equal to the charge for one day of hospital care. A copayment is made for each of the sixty-first through ninetieth days of inpatient care; it is equal to 25 percent of the deductible.

From the inception of the program until 1983, hospitals were reimbursed for their costs of providing care as defined by a complex set of regulations and formulas. They received estimated monthly payments that were adjusted at year end on the basis of a cost report submitted to the Health Care Financing Administration. Beginning in 1983, Medicare switched to a prospective payment system. A payment rate is assigned to approximately five hundred diagnosis-related groups (DRGs) according to the patient's age, sex, principal and secondary diagnosis, procedure performed (if any), and discharge status. Some hospitals (such as psychiatric, children's, and long-term care) are excluded from the prospective payment system and reimbursed under different arrangements.

Medicare Part B

Medicare Part B is financed 24 percent from premiums paid by enrollees and 76 percent from federal treasury funds. The monthly premium ($52 in 2002) is deducted directly from an enrollee's Social Security check.

Coverage includes physician care, physician-ordered supplies and durable medical equipment, services provided by some other categories of health professionals, and outpatient care.

Prior to 1992, physicians were paid fee-for-service on the basis of their "reasonable and customary" charges. In 1992, Medicare began making payments according to a resource-based relative value scale (RBRVS). Using this system, an index number is assigned to every physician encounter or procedure; it is based on the amount of work required, practice expenses, and malpractice insurance costs. To determine payment, the index number is multiplied by a standard conversion factor (or "going rate") that is established each year.

WELFARE INSURANCE (MEDICAID)

Medicaid was enacted in 1965 as Title 19 of the Social Security Act. The program finances provision of health care services to the poor. In a strict sense, Medicaid is not health insurance; rather, it is a welfare subsidy. Benefits are not earned but furnished to recipients in need.

In 2000, Medicaid covered forty-one million individuals. It is federally sponsored and supported (overseen by CMS) but state-administered. Fifty-seven percent of its funding is federal, 43 percent from the states.

States choose whether to have a Medicaid program; all but Arizona have decided to do so. Each state determines the need-based financial criteria that individuals must meet to be enrolled. Federal law mandates provision of certain minimum benefits, such as physician services, nonpreventive dental services, hospital inpatient care, hospital outpatient care, nursing home care, home health visits, and laboratory and X-ray services. Optional benefits can be offered at a state's discretion, including inpatient psychiatric care, optometrist care and eyeglasses, routine dental care, prescription drugs, and others. States determine utilization limits for both mandated and optional benefits and establish eligibility criteria, in addition to specifying the methods and rates for paying providers.

HEALTH MAINTENANCE ORGANIZATIONS

An HMO is a hybrid health care insurance and provider mechanism that offers a managed care plan. An HMO links together in one entity a health plan, hospitals, physicians, and other providers. Health plans can either contract with or own organizational providers; the former type of relationship is more common than the latter.

Health plans can secure professional services in three ways: (1) contract with individual physicians who remain independent and care for beneficiaries, in addition to other patients, in their offices (an IPA, or independent practice association, model of HMO); (2) contract with organized groups of physicians that either care for plan beneficiaries exclusively or do so in addition to other patients (group-model HMO); or (3) hire physicians as employees (staff-model HMO).

Hospitals can be closed-staff or open-staff. In a closed arrangement, only physicians who are employees of, or have contracted with, the health plan are medical staff members. In an open arrangement, health plan and other physicians are admitted to the medical staff.

The essential glue that binds the three parties together and structures their relationships with purchasers and beneficiaries consists of administration arrangements and economic incentives. They are designed to increase clinical quality and efficiency, manage utilization of services, and control costs through a number of mechanisms, such as:

- Limiting the type of benefits and services available to those deemed clinically and cost effective
- Restricting use of nonplan providers
- Paying a set rate to hospitals and physicians (per beneficiary, per month) for providing covered services irrespective of the amount and cost
- Assigning primary care physicians the task of gatekeeper to manage patients' use of hospital and specialist care
- Authorizing services before they are provided
- Implementing utilization and quality monitoring and review procedures

In 2000 approximately eighty-one million Americans, 30 percent of the population, received their health care through an HMO. Enrollment in these plans has increased from about five million in 1976 to more than eighty million in 2000. In 2000 there were 568 HMOs, up from 174 in 1976, a 226 percent increase over the period.

CHAPTER 4

Accounting Basics

OBJECTIVES

After completing this chapter, you will understand some key accounting concepts, terms, and principles that are employed to collect financial data and prepare financial statements.

A health care organization is an important social institution providing the community with essential services, but it is also a business. Engaging in economic activities (buying, producing, and selling), money moves into, through, and out of the organization. Decisions regarding the vision and strategy, types of programs and services offered, and quality of care provided all have financial implications. Revenues less expenses must be positive over the long run for a health care organization to remain viable. In short, money matters!

Accounting is the money-focused language of business. It records economic transactions and summarizes them in financial reports depicting an organization's financial performance and condition. An organization's basic financial statements are the revenue/expense summary, balance sheet, and statement of cash flows; reading and analyzing them is the focus of Chapters Five and Six. These statements are employed by external parties such as owners (shareholders and stakeholders), investors, lenders, donors, vendors, and regulators; and internal users such as boards, executives, and managers.

Whereas accounting records and reports past events, the discipline of financial management uses this information to monitor, analyze, plan, and make decisions; it looks forward into the organization's future.

The chapters in this book (with the exception of this and the following one, "Reading Financial Statements") focus on the governance-relevant aspects of financial management, not accounting. But to understand the information on which financial analysis, planning, and decision making are based, you must be familiar with key accounting concepts and terms.

ACCOUNTING PRINCIPLES

The recording and presenting of financial information is grounded in a set of standards: generally accepted accounting principles, or GAAP. They have evolved over many years and are influenced by such bodies as the Financial Accounting Standards Board (FASB) and the Government Accounting Standards Board (GASB). GAAP is designed to apply to all types of organizations; it is supplemented by industry-specific standards developed by the American Institute of Certified Public Accountants (AICPA). Additionally, in the health care industry accounting guidance is provided by the Principles and Practice Board of the Healthcare Financial Management Association (HFMA).

The thing to keep in mind is that GAAP must be followed. If it is not, auditors are unable to issue an unqualified opinion (the audit is addressed in Chapter Ten); this raises questions regarding whether financial statements can be relied upon by external parties (such as potential lenders) to analyze the organization's financial condition.

ACCOUNTING ENTITY

An accounting entity is that for which accounting information is collected and financial statements are prepared. Accounting entities do business, or are capable of doing so, on their own; they're what the nonaccountants among us call "organizations." A health system, hospital, nursing home, freestanding ambulatory surgery center, medical group, and home health agency are accounting entities. A hospital nursing *unit* is not. (If you don't buy this, try asking the chief financial officer for 3-West nursing unit's balance sheet.) Accounting entities need not necessarily be freestanding organizations or separately incorporated.

Accounting entities (from here out we'll call them organizations) come in many forms: sole proprietorships; corporations; partnerships; and a host of hybrids such as limited liability partnerships (LLPs), limited liability companies (LLCs), and professional corporations (PCs). They can be commercial (tax-paying), nonprofit (tax-exempt), or governmental.

You are likely responsible for governing a corporation that is:

- Formally chartered by the state
- Distinct and separate from its shareholders and stakeholders
- A so-called fictitious person (accorded many of the rights possessed by individuals)
- Has an unlimited life (transcending that of its directors, executives, and employees)
- Limits the liability of owners

This book focuses on nonprofit corporations providing health care services. However, what you learn here can be applied to most other organization types.

ACCOUNTING PERIOD

Economic transactions are recorded and reported for specific spans of time, called accounting periods. The base period is one year, which may be either calendar (January 1 through December 31) or fiscal (any consecutive twelve months). To facilitate timely reporting, analysis, and financial decision making, annual accounting periods are typically broken down into quarters and months.

MONETARY UNIT

Accounting is limited to recording and reporting only those organizational activities that can be quantified in monetary units. If something can't be expressed in dollars, it's beyond the realm of accounting and is not reflected in an organization's financial statements.

A lot of important things are left out, such as the increasing value of some types of assets (property, for instance); the effect of inflation; services donated by volunteers; the worth of the knowledge, skills, experience, and creativity of employees; and the value of an organization's climate and culture.

OBJECTIVITY

To record economic transactions in monetary terms, accountants require verifiable evidence: an invoice from a supplier, record of a service provided, bill sent to a patient, inventories of items in stock, or piece of equipment accompanied by proof of ownership. Tangible assets (facilities and equipment) are carried on an organization's books at their historical cost (which is objectively verifiable) rather than their estimated market value (which isn't).

ACCRUAL ACCOUNTING

GAAP requires that economic transactions be coupled within an accounting period; it's the foundational principle of accrual accounting. This is somewhat counterintuitive to nonaccountants, because it's unlike the way we keep our personal financial records (cash accounting).

In cash accounting, expenses are recognized when checks are written, and revenues are credited when checks are received—that is, when cash actually changes hands. This system is simple and totally adequate for a household or small business.

In accrual accounting, by contrast, revenues are recognized when they are earned—at the time services are provided—not when cash is received (from the patient, a health plan, Medicare, or Medicaid). Expenses are matched to the revenues they helped generate; revenues and expenses are thus matched. We return to this concept again and again in the chapters that follow.

MATERIALITY

The typical health care organization engages in hundreds of thousands, if not millions, of economic transactions during an accounting period. Reporting all of them individually would be totally overwhelming and not worth the cost, in terms of the value added to financial decision making. Thus accountants constantly make judgments and report at the level of detail that is deemed to be significant, relevant, and material to potential users of the information.

FULL DISCLOSURE AND TRANSPARENCY

Accounting information is employed by external parties to assess an organization's financial condition and decide whether they should invest in or lend money to it. Additionally, accounting reports are used internally to analyze, plan, and make decisions. Accordingly, financial statements must:

- Fairly reflect the organization's financial status, neither understating nor overstating its condition
- Disclose all material financial events and transactions and not avoid unpleasant circumstances
- Be easily understood by a knowledgeable reader, not veiled in unnecessary complexity

CONSERVATISM, CONSISTENCY, AND COMPARABILITY

The process of recording and reporting financial transactions is designed to be conservative. For example, accountants typically recognize good news only when it actually happens and report bad news if it is likely to occur; and, when in doubt, err on the side of undervaluing assets and overvaluing obligations.

To be useful, financial reporting must be consistent; that is, the same type of transaction must be recorded and reported in identical ways across accounting periods. Absent this, financial statements are not standardized over time.

Consistency focuses on a given organization over time; comparability deals with standardization across organizations. It requires the same accounting methods and procedures (that is, application of GAAP) to be employed to record and report financial transactions of all like-type organizations (for instance, all hospitals). Otherwise, the financial statements of similar organizations would be idiosyncratic.

ACCOUNTING VALUE

The accounting value of an organizational asset or liability is determined by applying GAAP, and it may differ significantly from the actual worth. For example:

- As discussed more fully later in this chapter, facilities and equipment are recorded or reported at their historical cost, not current market value.
- Billed patient charges are adjusted to reflect the estimated amount that will actually be collected.
- An organization's worth is an accounting estimate rather than what might actually remain if the business were sold and all liabilities settled.

So keep in mind that accounting entries reflect, but do not necessarily equal, the market value of an asset or liability.

ACCOUNTING EQUATION

Financial "ground zero" is the accounting equation, expressed as:

$$\text{Assets} = \text{Liabilities} + \text{Owners equity}$$

Assets are what an organization *owns*. Liabilities are what an organization *owes*. Owners equity is what an organization is *worth*.

Assets

Assets are the monetary value of what an organization possesses, such as:

- Cash and cash equivalents, such as money in savings accounts and certificates of deposit (CDs)
- Accounts receivable: essentially IOUs for services that have been provided but not yet paid by patients, health plans, HMOs, Medicare, and Medicaid
- Inventory: supplies held to provide patient care services (such as drugs and food)
- Fixed assets: property, plant, and equipment

Liabilities

Liabilities are the monetary value of what's owed—claims against the organization by creditors, such as:

- Accounts payable: obligations to external parties for goods and services received
- Accrued wages, salaries, and benefits: what the organization owes for work that has been performed by employees
- Long-term debt (liabilities that will be settled more than one year in the future), including the principal owed on mortgages and bonds

Owners equity

Owners equity is the organization's worth when liabilities are subtracted from total assets. It is a product of transposing the accounting equation:

$$\text{Assets} = \text{Liabilities} + \text{Owners equity}$$
$$\text{Owners equity} = \text{Assets} - \text{Liabilities}$$

Think of it this way: if a hospital sold all of its assets for the value carried on its books and used the proceeds to pay off all debts, what's left would be owners equity. Owners equity belongs to the organization's "owners" (stockholders in a commercial corporation, stakeholders in a nonprofit). In nonprofit organizations, the term used for owners equity is *net assets*. The term *owners equity* is employed throughout the book because we feel it is more descriptive.

All organizations could keep their books using only three accounts, one for each component of the accounting equation: assets, liabilities, and owners equity. However, this would not yield enough information to assess financial condition, or plan and make decisions. Accordingly, other accounts are created. Two of the most important are *revenues* and *expenses*. Revenues increase the value of an organization, and expenses decrease it; the difference between them is *net income* (profit). In the financial statements of nonprofit health care organizations, the term *excess of revenues over expenses* is often used instead of net income.

REVENUES

Revenues are the flow of assets into the organization from the sale of goods and services. There are two types: operating and nonoperating.

Operating revenues are generated by activities closely related to an organization's core mission; for a hospital, providing health care services. Thus operating revenues include what the organization earns by providing patient services, and those that come from related activities such as operating a cafeteria, parking lot, and gift shop.

Nonoperating revenues are derived from activities not closely tied to the provision of patient care, such as earnings from financial investments and unrelated business income from a restaurant, hotel, or consulting firm. There is a broad range of discretion regarding what constitutes operating and nonoperating revenues.

Keep in mind that all revenues are recorded (booked) when they are earned, not when payment in cash is actually received.

EXPENSES

Expenses are the cost of resources consumed in the process of generating revenues during an accounting period. They are matched to revenues generated, not when paid in cash.

Essentials of Health Care Organization Finance

Expenses include the obvious stuff, discussed previously: employee salaries and benefits, cost of supplies, purchased services, and insurance premiums. One item included as an expense on an organization's books is *depreciation.*

Because of the requirements of accrual accounting, resources consumed are matched with revenues earned in the same period. When a fixed asset (say, a piece of radiology equipment) is purchased, the manufacturer is paid and cash flows out of the organization. It would be unreasonable to expense the full cost of this equipment in the accounting period when it was purchased. Matching would not be achieved; the costs are booked in one period, but the equipment is used to generate revenues throughout its useful life, over many years. Depreciation is an accounting convention and technique employed to spread the cost of long-lived assets (such as plant and equipment) over the period of time in which they are actually used to generate revenues. Exhibit 4.1 presents the concept graphically.

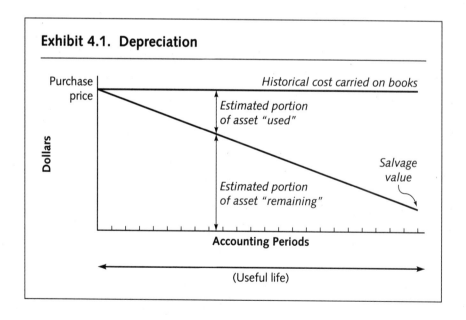

Exhibit 4.1. Depreciation

A fixed asset, such as that piece of radiology equipment, is carried on an organization's books at its historical cost (purchase price plus the cost of delivery and installation). The asset's useful life and salvage value are estimated. The portion of the asset's total cost expensed in a particular accounting period is calculated as:

$$\begin{array}{c}\text{depreciation}\\\text{expense in an}\\\text{accounting}\\\text{period}\end{array} = \frac{\text{purchase price} - \text{estimated salvage value}}{\begin{array}{c}\text{estimated useful}\\\text{life of the asset}\\\text{(years)}\end{array}}$$

An illustration is in Exhibit 4.2.

Exhibit 4.2. Illustrative Depreciation Calculation

Equipment purchase price (plus cost of shipping and installation)	$400,000
Estimated salvage value (at end of useful life)	–$50,000
Depreciable value	$350,000
Estimated useful life	5 years
Annual depreciation ($350,000 divided by 5 years)	$70,000

SUMMARY

This chapter has laid out some key accounting concepts. Exhibit 4.3 conveys the big picture and some important relationships:

• Health care organizations, in addition to being social institutions, are business entities and must function accordingly.

• The economic events, activities, and transactions in which they engage during an accounting period are recorded in the organization's books, following GAAP.

• These books are used by accountants to prepare financial statements: revenue/expense summary, balance sheet, and statement of cash flows.

• Such statements are used by external parties to assess an organization's financial condition and to make lending and investment decisions. They are also employed by internal users such as executives and boards to analyze, plan, make decisions, and control operations.

In the next two chapters, we turn to reading financial statements, analyzing them, and the board's role of overseeing a health care organization's financial performance and condition.

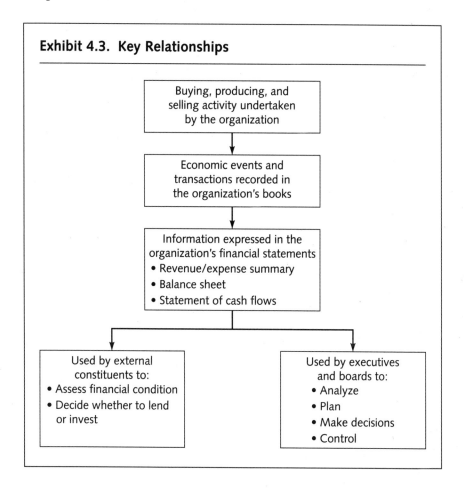

Exhibit 4.3. Key Relationships

Buying, producing, and selling activity undertaken by the organization

Economic events and transactions recorded in the organization's books

Information expressed in the organization's financial statements
• Revenue/expense summary
• Balance sheet
• Statement of cash flows

Used by external constituents to:
• Assess financial condition
• Decide whether to lend or invest

Used by executives and boards to:
• Analyze
• Plan
• Make decisions
• Control

CHAPTER 5

Reading Financial Statements

OBJECTIVES

After completing this chapter, you will:

- Be able to read and interpret key financial statements that reflect your organization's financial status
- Become familiar with additional accounting concepts and principles

I f accounting is the monetary language of business, then its foundational documents are the revenue/expense summary, balance sheet, and statement of cash flows. Information collected by accountants about an organization's economic activities is summarized and portrayed in them.

Illustrative Financial Statements You Will Be Seeing Here

Welcome to E. Polley Francis Hospital (EPFH), a fictitious illustration employed in this and the following chapters. EPFH is a nonprofit, short-term, general hospital that is freestanding (not part of a system).

    EPFH's financial statements have been simplified to make learning to read them easy. Additionally, we have inserted some instructional aids (such

---

(Continued)

as bold and italicized text, indentations, and equal signs) that you won't find on traditionally prepared statements.

Appendix A of this book contains sets of financial statements similar to the ones you are likely to see in your boardroom.

Financial statements should be compiled following GAAP (generally accepted accounting principles). Their structure and format is standardized but varies somewhat by type of industry and organization.

Each financial statement has a header, in three parts:

E. Polley Francis Hospital ← (1)
Balance Sheet ← (2)
< December 31, 2006 > ← (3)

1. *The name of the business entity.* This can be a single organization or a collection of them (a "consolidated financial statement")

2. *The type of statement* (revenue/expense summary, balance sheet, or statement of cash flows)

3. *The date of the statement or accounting period it covers.* The balance sheet reports an organization's financial status at a point in time; the revenue/expense summary and statement of cash flows cover an accounting period (month, quarter, or year).

Other than for very small organizations, figures are expressed in thousands of dollars rounded to the nearest thousand. Thus the amount $1,352,886 becomes $1,353. Note that in illustrative financial statements, figures are expressed in '000s (dropping the last three zeros); in text, the full amount in dollars is used.

REVENUE/EXPENSE SUMMARY

The most basic questions that can be asked about an organization's finances are: How much revenue was earned? What were its expenses? Did it produce a profit or incur a loss? The revenue/expense summary, shown in Exhibit 5.1

Essentials of Health Care Organization Finance

You've Been Here Before

Ask someone if he or she has prepared financial statements, and the reply is likely to be, "Heck no, I'm not an accountant." Well, have you ever applied for a home mortgage? Many of us have. At the time, you provided the lender with information about your financial condition by completing two forms. Although not labeled as such, one was a balance sheet, listing what you own and what you owe (the difference being your net worth). The other was a revenue/expense summary, detailing your annual monetary inflow, outflow, and the difference between them (your net income).

Exhibit 5.1. E. Polley Francis Hospital's Revenue/Expense Summary for Period Ending December 31, 2006

Revenues (operations)		
Net patient revenues		$323,100
Other revenues		$17,600
	Total revenues =	$340,700
Expenses (operations)		
Salaries and benefits		$158,000
Supplies and other		$138,500
Depreciation		$20,667
Interest expense		$3,400
Provision for uncollectables		$7,300
	Total expenses =	$327,867
	Net income from operations =	$12,833
	Net nonoperating income =	$8,915
Net income		$21,748

(also called the "income statement" or "statement of operations" in commercial corporations), gives the answers. It is prepared for an accounting period (month, quarter, or year) and portrays revenues earned, expenses incurred, and net income (profit) generated during the period, where:

$$\text{Net income} = \text{Revenues} - \text{Expenses}$$

The revenue/expense summary is the least standardized financial statement; all such statements show the basics, but subcategories and detail vary from organization to organization.

Revenue from Operations

The focus is revenues earned from activities directly related to, or closely associated with, an organization's core mission; for E. Polley Francis Hospital (EPFH), it is the provision of health care services.

Recall that, because accrual accounting is employed, revenues are recorded in the accounting period when they are earned, not when cash is actually received. EPFH shows annual (January 1 through December 31, 2006) total revenues from operations of $340,700,000.

Net patient revenues of EPFH were $323,100,000. This is money earned from the core business of providing patient services.

Revenues are stated in net terms. It is an estimate of what an organization expects to be paid (or reimbursed), not necessarily the full charges billed. This is important because there is generally a substantial difference between list price (billed charges) and ultimate cash receipts. Here are several illustrations:

• Medicare (as discussed in Chapter Three) pays a flat DRG rate for inpatient care, not the listed charges for each individual service provided to a patient during a stay.

• Most health plans negotiate discounts from full charges for services provided to their beneficiaries.

• HMOs might pay a flat rate for hospital care per enrollee per month, irrespective of how many services were furnished.

Essentials of Health Care Organization Finance

Additionally, net patient revenues are calculated less charges associated with providing services to those, who at the time they received them, are not expected to pay; this is *charity care.*

All of these are *deductions* from revenues; accordingly, accountants and financial managers must estimate them. This is done on the basis of historical data, examining reimbursement regulations and contract terms, which all require making a number of assumptions. The reasonableness and accuracy of these estimates have a significant impact on the statement of operating revenues, and eventually net income (profits). An underestimate inflates revenues and artificially boosts an organization's financial health; an overestimate deflates revenues and makes an organization appear to be in worse financial shape than it actually is.

EPFH shows *other operating revenue* of $17,600,000. The sources are activities indirectly related to the organization's core mission, such as running a cafeteria, gift shop, or parking lot. Also included are unrestricted donations.

Operating Expenses

This section reflects the value of resources used to produce operating revenues earned during the accounting period.

EPFH breaks down operating expenses into five categories (you may see different ones in the revenue/expense summary for your organization): salaries and benefits, supplies and other, depreciation, interest expenses, and provision for uncollectables. The first two are self-explanatory; we focus attention on the remaining three.

Remember (from Chapter Four) that property, plant, and equipment are carried on an organization's books at their historical cost. *Depreciation* matches the cost of these long-lived assets to the revenues they helped generate. EPFH shows depreciation of $20,667,000; this is the accounting value of the portion of fixed assets expensed (and matched to revenues generated) during the period.

EPFH had *interest expenses* of $3,400,000, the amount paid or owed to lenders for both short-term and long-term debt during the accounting period. In most health care organizations, the largest portion is interest expense on bonds.

The last line is *provision for uncollectables* ($7,300,000), or bad debt. This reflects revenues generated during the accounting period the organization estimates will not be paid due to the risk of extending credit.

All totaled, EPFH had *operating expenses* of $327,867,000; this is its cost of doing business during the accounting period.

Bottom of the Page

EPFH shows a *net income from operations* of $12,833,000:

Net operating income		Operating revenues		Operating expenses
$12,833,000	=	$340,700,000	–	$327,867,000

This is the profit from EPFH's core business of providing health care services.

Most organizations engage in some activities not related to their core mission. EPFH's *net nonoperating income* (nonoperating revenues less non-operating expenses, not shown on the statement) from such endeavors is $8,915,000. Illustrative sources are (1) strictly financial investments, (2) consulting services provided to other organizations, (3) unrelated business income (from an owned hotel, restaurant, or sports club), and (4) gains or losses from the sale of fixed assets.

Net income (profit, or margin; a number of terms are used) is the difference between an organization's total revenues and total expenses during the accounting period; it is also referred to as *the bottom line*. For EPFH, it's $21,748,000. Net income is not cash in the bank, due to accrual accounting. Nor is it what the organization is worth (a concept addressed in the next section). It's the net increase in an organization's value during the accounting period from conducting business.

BALANCE SHEET

A balance sheet is a snapshot of an organization's financial status at a specific point in time; for EPFH (Exhibit 5.2), it is at midnight on December 31, 2006. The balance sheet puts flesh on the accounting equation:

Assets = Liabilities + Owners equity

Exhibit 5.2. E. Polley Francis Hospital's Balance Sheet for December 31, 2006

Assets		Liabilities	
Current assets		**Current liabilities**	
Cash and marketable securities	$38,200	Payroll accruals	$17,400
Accounts receivable (net)	$67,900	Accounts payable	$29,900
Inventories	$6,600	Current portion of long-term debt	$4,300
Prepaid and other	$1,100	Payable to agencies	$17,180
Total current assets =	$113,800	Total current liabilities =	$68,780
Noncurrent assets		Long-term debt	$48,800
Long-term investments	$94,595	Total liabilities =	$117,580
Property, plant, and equipment	$368,420		
(Less) accumulated depreciation	–$208,600		
		Owners equity	$250,635
Total noncurrent assets =	$254,415		
Total assets =	$368,215	Total liabilities and owners equity =	$368,215

Balance sheets have "left hand" and "right hand" sides: assets are on the left, liabilities and owners equity are on the right. The totals must balance (both sides must be equal). The assets held by an organization (what it owns) must equal liabilities (what it owes) plus owners equity (what it is worth).

Left Side

Assets are what the organization owns, expressed in monetary terms. This includes cash, inventory, facilities, and equipment. Assets are listed on the balance sheet in decreasing order of liquidity. For example, current assets are more liquid than noncurrent assets; within current assets, marketable securities can be converted into cash more quickly than inventory.

The balance sheet portrays two broad categories of assets: current and noncurrent. The total for EPFH is $368,215,000.

Current assets are relatively liquid—cash per se or assets intended to be converted into cash within one year during the normal course of business. EPFH shows current assets of $113,800,000, which include:

- *Cash* (and cash equivalents) such as petty cash, money held in checking and bank accounts, and certificates of deposit. Also included here (but sometimes broken out as separate lines) are marketable securities—short-term and readily marketable financial instruments such as commercial paper and treasury bills.

- *Net accounts receivable* represent a debt owed to the organization for services it has provided to patients (at their estimated collection value) that has yet to be paid.

- *Inventories* are the amount paid for such things as drugs, supplies, and disposables that are intended to be used within one year.

- *Prepaid* items are assets of the organization that have been paid in advance, such as insurance and rent on equipment or facilities.

- *Other* is a catch-all category for miscellaneous minor assets that are not material enough to warrant a separate line on the balance sheet.

Noncurrent assets are those not intended to be converted into cash within one year during the normal course of business. For EPFH, they are $254,415,000 and include:

- *Long-term investments,* financial assets held by an organization, including stocks and bonds. These investments are considered long-term because of their intended use (holding them for more than one year), even though most of them can be converted to cash in a shorter time period.
- *Property, plant, and equipment* (also called fixed assets or PPE), carried on the books at their historical cost.
- *Accumulated depreciation.* Since fixed assets are recorded at their historical cost, their accounting worth in the present period must be adjusted for depreciation; this line of the balance sheet does so. EPFH shows accumulated depreciation of $208,600,000; this is the total amount of depreciation expense incurred in the present and past accounting periods for fixed assets the organization still owns. It is deducted from the historical cost of property, plant, and equipment; for EPFH, this is $368,420,000. You may run across the term *book value.* This is the historical cost of fixed assets the organization still owns minus accumulated depreciation expensed in the current and past accounting periods—that is, the remaining accounting value of fixed assets. EPFH's book value of fixed assets is $159,820,000 ($368,420,000 less $208,600,000).

EPFH's *total assets,* the value of what it owns, are $368,215,000.

Right Side

The right-hand side of a balance sheet is composed of liabilities (what the organization owes to creditors) plus owners equity (what the organization is worth). In nonprofits and governmental agencies owners equity is labeled "net assets." Regardless of the term used, the organization's worth is found on the lower right-hand side of the balance sheet.

Liabilities are what is owed to outside parties (lenders and extenders of credit). There are two types: current and long-term.

Current liabilities are claims that, in the normal course of business, will be settled in less than one year; they are parallel to current assets, on the left-hand side of the balance sheet, which will be received in one year. EPFH's balance sheet has four categories of them (other organizations may list more):

1. *Payroll accruals* ($17,400,000) include salaries, wages, benefits, and payroll taxes (such as Social Security) that have been incurred but not yet paid in cash.

2. *Accounts payable* ($29,900,000), also referred to as trade payables, are amounts owed to vendors for services, supplies, and equipment.

3. *Current portions of long-term debt* ($4,300,000) include principal payments on mortgages and bonds due within one year.

4. *Payables to agencies.* In some cases, health care organizations receive interim payments from payors (such as health plans, Medicare, and Medicaid) based on estimates of what they owe for services provided to their beneficiaries. Usually, these periodic reimbursements are different (either more or less) from what payors actually owe. This line on the balance sheet indicates that EPFH estimates, when everything is settled, it will owe payors $17,180,000.

EPFH's balance sheet shows total current liabilities of $68,780,000.

Long-term debt, sometimes labeled "noncurrent liabilities," is the amount an organization owes on loans that have maturities greater than one year; typically this is for mortgages, bonds, and capital lease obligations. We return to this part of the balance sheet in Chapter Eight, dealing with an

---

Working Capital

You are likely to hear the term *working capital*. It is calculated here for EPFH as:

Working capital		Current assets		Current liabilities
$45,020,000	=	$113,800,000	−	$68,780,000

This is a reflection of the organization's liquidity; how much current assets exceed or are less than current liabilities. Phrased as a question, Does the organization have adequate current assets (cash or resources easily convertible into it) to pay obligations that will come due within the next year? If it does not, the organization has a liquidity problem.

Essentials of Health Care Organization Finance

organization's capital structure, creditworthiness, and long-term debt financing. EPFH has long-term debt of $48,800,000.

Owners equity is what an organization is worth. It's a product of transposing the accounting equation introduced in Chapter Four. Using EPFH's figures, here is the calculation:

Owners equity		Total assets		Total liabilities
$250,635,000	=	$368,215,000	−	$117,580,000

Owners equity is what would remain if EPFH sold all its assets at their accounting value as stated on its balance sheet and paid off all liabilities (both short-term and long-term).

Why is owners equity on the right-hand side of the balance sheet? There are two answers. First, it must be, to make the balance sheet balance. Second, and a far better response: it's a claim that owners (stockholders or stakeholders) have on the organization; it is parallel to liabilities, claims that lenders have on the organization's assets.

In nonprofits, owners equity is created in a number of ways:

- Contributions and grants received when the organization was founded
- In health care systems, funds transferred into the organization by a parent entity
- Sale of stock in commercial corporations
- Tax levy transfers into the organization
- Most important, accumulation of profit (net income) over the years

EPFH's owners equity is shown on the balance sheet as $250,635,000.

Summary

The balance sheet (see Exhibit 5.3) is a picture of an organization's financial condition at a particular point in time. It's a portrayal of the accounting equation:

$$\text{Assets} = \text{Liabilities} + \text{Owners equity}$$

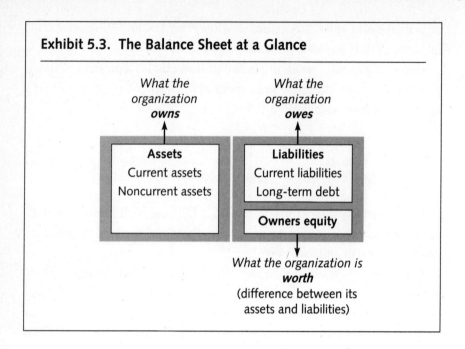

Exhibit 5.3. The Balance Sheet at a Glance

What the organization **owns**

What the organization **owes**

Assets
Current assets
Noncurrent assets

Liabilities
Current liabilities
Long-term debt

Owners equity

What the organization is **worth**
(difference between its assets and liabilities)

Assets are on the left-hand side; liabilities and owners equity are on the right. Assets are what an organization owns. Liabilities, both current and long-term, are what an organization owes to creditors. Owners equity, the difference between total assets and total liabilities, is what an organization is worth.

STATEMENT OF CASH FLOWS

Finance professionals often say, "cash is king." The reason: it is the only thing an organization can actually spend. If an organization doesn't have (or is chronically short of) cash, it won't be in business for long. Virtually all business transactions are eventually settled by cash inflows to, or outflows from, the organization. Cash is an organization's most basic fuel, and it's not advisable to run on empty!

The balance sheet shows (as a current asset) the amount of cash on hand at a specific point in time. This is important information, but incomplete.

Essentials of Health Care Organization Finance

Did cash increase or decrease during the accounting period? Where did it come from? How was it used? The statement of cash flows (Exhibit 5.4) answers these questions.

Exhibit 5.4. E. Polley Francis Hospital's Statement of Cash Flows

Net cash flow from operating activities	$36,415
Net cash flow from investing activities	−$31,015
Net cash flow from financing activities	−$3,600
Increase (decrease) in cash =	$1,800
Beginning cash balance	$36,400
Ending cash balance	$38,200

There are three sources and uses of cash: operating activities, investing activities, and financing activities.

Operating activities show the cash increase or decrease related to an organization's core mission; for health care organizations, this is provision of patient services. Operations must ultimately be the source of cash for an organization to survive and thrive; absent this, it has to rely on donations and tax contributions. EPFH has a *net cash flow from operations* of $36,415,000.

Investing activities show the increase or decrease in cash that is due to investing in assets such as facilities and equipment. EPFH's investing activities decreased cash by $31,015,000.

Financing activities show uses of cash: to pay down principal on the organization's long-term debt, and receipt of cash when long-term debt proceeds or owner contributions (donations) are received. EPFH's financing activities decreased cash by $3,600,000.

EPFH's net increase in cash from operating, investing, and financing activity was $1,800,000. When this is added to cash on hand at the beginning of the accounting period ($36,400,000), its *ending cash balance* is $38,200,000.

IN THE BOARDROOM

➤ The type and format of financial information your board requires to govern differs from what executives need to manage. Many boards receive financial statements that are good for managing but poor for governing. They may be too detailed and too complex and contain a lot of information that is not relevant to the board in doing its job. For board use, you may want to consider asking that financial statements be prepared in the format presented here (which would not be acceptable for external use) so they are easier to read and interpret: stripped down, with use of equal signs, indentations, and highlights.

➤ Whether the reports are board-friendly or "typical," obtain copies of your organization's revenue/expense summary, balance sheet, and statement of cash flows. Using what you have learned in this chapter, begin reading. Go over each statement section by section, line by line. Recall that the statements you see will be a bit different from the ones we've used here as illustrations. If you have questions (quite likely if you're a non-accountant), make an appointment with the CFO for a personal tutorial. Expect the CFO to answer your questions in a straightforward, clear, and intelligible way.

➤ Your board should receive financial statements at least quarterly, included in the agenda book and distributed at least one week prior to meetings. We think it's critical that the finance committee carefully review them prior to the board meeting and develop a set of comments and questions; these can either be attached to the statements in the agenda book or reviewed at the meeting. You should expect adequate time to be devoted at the meeting for directors to discuss these statements and deliberate their implications for the organization's financial condition, now and in the future.

➤ General questions you may want to ask:

Are your organization's financial statements prepared in accordance with GAAP? If not, why not? This may seem too obvious, but it is so important that it must be asked.

Essentials of Health Care Organization Finance

If you are a director of a health care organization composed of multiple business entities, is your board given consolidated financial statements (for the system) in addition to component business entities? If not, it's impossible to get a feel for the financial condition of the corporation as a whole.

➤ Questions regarding the revenue/expense summary that you might want to ask:

Who are your organization's major payors? What proportion of net patient revenues is derived from Medicare, Medicaid, other governmental programs, health plans (Blue Cross and commercial), health maintenance organizations, and private (customer out-of-pocket) pay? How has the mix changed over the past three years?

What is the percentage of deductions subtracted from gross patient revenues to produce net patient revenues? How accurately have these deductions been estimated over the past five years? Recognize that inaccurate estimates pose a significant risk because they result in overestimating or underestimating net revenues and hence profits.

How much bad debt did your organization incur last year? Has it been increasing or decreasing over time? What are your organization's policies regarding when and how credit is extended?

How much charity care did your organization provide last year? What has been the trend? What is your organization's policy regarding provision of charity care?

What is included in the line for other revenue? Historically, what has been the variability of such revenues across accounting periods?

What is included in net nonoperating income? How dependent is the organization on this source of income?

➤ Questions regarding the balance sheet that you might want to ask:

How much working capital (current assets less current liabilities) does your organization have? How has it changed over the last five years?

What are the largest categories of inventory? How are they managed? For example, does your organization have a just-in-time system in place? Does it belong to a group purchasing organization?

How are long-term investments deployed and managed (and by whom)? Does your board have an investment policy and objectives (regarding such things as yields and fees)?

What is the long-term trend in owners equity? Has it been increasing or decreasing over time?

➤ Questions regarding the cash flow statement that you might want to ask:

The big one: Does your organization have a net positive cash flow from operations? What has been the trend over the last three years?

During the last three years, has your organization ever been late in making principal payments on its long-term debt?

➤ If your organization has done a bond financing in the last three years, request a copy of the bond document. This is a terrific source of information regarding your organization's financial condition.

CHAPTER 6

Analyzing Financial Statements and Overseeing Financial Performance

OBJECTIVES

After completing this chapter, you will be able to:

- Use horizontal, vertical, and ratio techniques to analyze your organization's financial statements
- Work with fellow directors to oversee your organization's financial performance and condition

In this chapter, we move from accounting (recording and reporting financial transactions) to managerial finance, using this information to assess, plan, and make decisions. Financial analysis helps to ask and answer some key questions. How financially healthy is an organization? If there are problems, what caused them? What should be done about the situation? The board is responsible for asking the first two questions. Management is responsible for having an answer to the third.

With the revenue/expense summary and balance sheet, there are a number of relationships that can be analyzed. We focus on a few illustrations to introduce you to the area of financial statement analysis.

There are three types of analysis: horizontal, vertical, and ratio. Each has its distinctive uses, strengths, and weaknesses. No one figure, percentage, statistic, or ratio is sufficient taken alone. To paint a complete picture and draw meaningful inferences, they must be used in combination. Additionally, financial analyses produce diagnostic measures; they don't necessarily indicate why something is the way it is, or what should be done if all is not right.

Illustrative financial statements for E. Polley Francis Hospital (see Exhibits 6.1, 6.2, and 6.3) are the same as those used in Chapter Five; here they portray two years of information—the current (2006, employed in Chapter Five) and immediately preceding (2005) accounting periods.

Exhibit 6.1. E. Polley Francis Hospital's Revenue/Expense Summary for Years Ending 2006 and 2005

	Year 2006	Year 2005
Revenues (operations)		
Net patient revenues	$323,100	$303,300
Other revenues	$17,600	$17,700
Total revenues =	$340,700	$321,000
Expenses (operations)		
Salaries and benefits	$158,000	$150,000
Supplies and other	$138,500	$129,000
Depreciation	$20,667	$19,033
Interest expense	$3,400	$3,500
Provision for uncollectables	$7,300	$7,800
Total expenses =	$327,867	$309,333
Net income from operations =	$12,833	$11,667
Net nonoperating income =	$8,915	$8,344
Net income	$21,748	$20,011

Exhibit 6.2. E. Polley Francis Hospital's Balance Sheet for December 31, 2006, and December 31, 2005

	Year 2006	Year 2005
Assets		
Current assets		
Cash and marketable securities	$38,200	$36,400
Accounts receivable (net)	$67,900	$65,400
Inventories	$6,600	$6,700
Prepaid and other	$1,100	$1,300
Total current assets =	$113,800	$109,800
Noncurrent assets		
Long-term investments	$94,595	$89,200
Property, plant, and equipment	$368,420	$342,800
(Less) accumulated depreciation	-$208,600	-$189,200
Total noncurrent assets =	$254,415	$242,800
Total assets =	**$368,215**	**$352,600**
Liabilities		
Current liabilities		
Payroll accruals	$17,400	$16,000
Accounts payable	$29,900	$25,000
Current portion of long-term debt	$4,300	$4,100
Payables, agencies	$17,180	$27,280
Total current liabilities =	$68,780	$72,380
Long-term debt	$48,800	$52,600
Total liabilities =	$117,580	$124,980
Owners equity (net assets)	$250,635	$227,620
Total liabilities and owners equity =	**$368,215**	**$352,600**

Exhibit 6.3. E. Polley Francis Hospital's Statement of Cash Flows for Years Ending December 31, 2006 and 2005

	Year 2006	Year 2005
Net cash flow from operating activities	$36,415	$40,044
Net cash flow from investing activities	–$31,015	–$34,644
Net cash flow from financing activities	–$3,600	–$3,500
Increase (decrease) in cash =	$1,800	$1,900
Beginning cash balance	$36,400	$34,500
Ending cash balance	$38,200	$36,400

HORIZONTAL AND VERTICAL ANALYSES

Horizontal analysis focuses on individual lines in financial statements. Increases and decreases across two or more accounting periods are calculated. Exhibit 6.4 portrays illustrative horizontal analyses of EPFH's revenue/expense summary and balance sheet.

There are no standards or benchmarks here, other than an organization's own past performance; this is a limitation of the approach. It is a great tool for identifying changes or trends and asking: Are they favorable or unfavorable? What caused them? What are the implications, both short-term and long-term? Horizontal analysis, and for that matter the underlying financial statements, don't give answers; one has to dig deeper into both finances and operations.

The strength of horizontal analysis is that it's easy to do, focuses attention on changes, and identifies things that should be moving together (for example, net revenue and net income) but may not be. The weaknesses of this type of analysis are that it's coarse, it does not take into account inflation or changes in an organization's size or volume over time, and it is not suitable for comparison with other organizations. Horizontal analysis can be beefed up by plotting trends and portraying them graphically, over a number of accounting periods.

Exhibit 6.4. E. Polley Francis Hospital: Illustrative Horizontal Financial Statement Analysis

	Year 2006	Year 2005	Increase/ (decrease) 2005–2006	Percentage change 2005–2006
Revenue/expense summary				
Net patient revenues	$323,100	$303,300	$19,800	6.5%
Total revenues	$340,700	$321,000	$19,700	6.1%
Salaries and benefits	$158,000	$150,000	$8,000	5.3%
Total expenses	$327,867	$309,333	$18,534	6.0%
Net income from operations	$12,833	$11,667	$1,166	10.0%
Net nonoperating income	$8,915	$8,344	$571	6.8%
Net income	$21,748	$20,011	$1,737	8.7%
Balance sheet				
Net accounts receivable	$67,900	$65,400	$2,500	3.8%
Total current assets	$113,800	$109,800	$4,000	3.6%
Total noncurrent assets	$254,415	$242,800	$11,615	4.8%
Total current liablities	$68,780	$72,380	–$3,600	–5.0%
Long-term debt	$48,800	$52,600	–$3,800	–7.2%
Total liabilities	$117,580	$124,980	–$7,400	–5.9%
Owners equity	$250,635	$227,620	$23,015	10.1%

Vertical analysis focuses on two lines of a financial statement (in a single accounting period), expressing one as a percentage of the other. This standardizes for changes in size or volume over time and adjusts for differences between organizations (in comparative analyses). Unlike horizontal analysis, measures are relative, rather than absolute. Exhibit 6.5 depicts some illustrative vertical analyses for EPFH.

Exhibit 6.5. E. Polley Francis Hospital: Illustrative Vertical Financial Statement Analysis

		Year 2006	Year 2005
Revenue/expense summary			
Net patient revenues		$323,100	$303,300
Total revenues		$340,700	$321,000
	Percentage =	94.8%	94.5%
Net income from operations		$12,833	$11,667
Total revenues		$340,700	$321,000
	Percentage =	3.8%	3.6%
Net income		$21,748	$20,011
Total revenue		$340,700	$321,000
	Percentage =	6.4%	6.2%
Balance sheet			
Current assets		$113,800	$109,800
Total assets		$368,215	$352,600
	Percentage =	30.9%	31.1%
Current liabilities		$68,780	$72,380
Total assets		$368,215	$352,600
	Percentage =	18.7%	20.5%
Long-term debt		$48,800	$52,600
Total assets		$368,215	$352,600
	Percentage =	13.3%	14.9%

Essentials of Health Care Organization Finance

The first line for each calculation is the numerator, and the second line is the denominator. For example, net patient revenues in 2006 is 94.8 percent of total revenues: ($323,100,000 / $340,700,000) × 100 = 94.8%. As with horizontal analysis, it's useful to plot trends graphically over multiple accounting periods.

RATIO ANALYSIS

The concept and calculation of a financial ratio is simple: one number is divided by another (and sometimes multiplied by 100 to produce a percentage).

$$\frac{\text{Numerator}}{\text{Denominator}} = \text{RATIO}$$

The numerator and denominator can be a single figure or a combination of them; they might be drawn from one or several financial statements.

There are hundreds of financial ratios, many of which have been developed for specific industries and particular organizational types. Ratios are the indicators most frequently employed by outsiders (such as bond rating and insurance agencies, lenders, and investors) to assess an organization's financial condition and by insiders (boards and executives) to analyze, plan, and make decisions. The reason is their calculation is standardized, and benchmarks are available that can be employed to assess an organization's financial condition and make comparisons with like-type institutions.

There are four types of financial ratio: liquidity, profitability, capital structure, and activity. Each takes its own look at an organization.

The sections that follow:

- Introduce some commonly used and representative ratios
- Show how they are calculated
- Illustrate them from EPFH's financial statements
- Briefly discuss what each ratio means and its implications
- Compare EPFH's ratios to benchmarks

Liquidity Ratios

Liquidity ratios measure an organization's ability to meet its short-term obligations (current liabilities) with its available resources (current assets). Most organizations get into financial trouble because of liquidity problems—a lack of cash to pay debts as they come due.

The *current ratio* is the most basic measure of liquidity. It's calculated as:

$$\frac{\text{Current assets}}{\text{Current liabilities}}$$

for EPFH:

$$\frac{\$113,800,000}{\$68,780,000} = 1.65$$

Both the numerator and denominator are taken from the balance sheet. This ratio measures how many times current liabilities can be paid with (or covered by) current assets. Current assets are considered "lazy" because they are not invested in producing services and thus don't generate revenues. Organizations want to hold as few of them as absolutely necessary, while maintaining the ability to meet short-term obligations as they come due.

EPFH's current ratio is 1.65, indicating that for every dollar of current liabilities the hospital has $1.65 in current assets. The benchmark is 2.0; that is, current assets should be about twice current liabilities. EPFH is below this benchmark, indicating that it may be experiencing liquidity problems. A finer-grained analysis would be needed to detect whether this is the case. "Drilling down" requires calculating additional ratios: days of cash on hand and days in accounts receivable.

From a lender's perspective, values of the current ratio above the benchmark and trends upward are desirable; values below the benchmark and trends headed downward are undesirable.

Essentials of Health Care Organization Finance

Days of cash on hand measures the number of days an organization can meet its average daily operating cash outlays with available cash and financial investments. It's typically calculated as:

$$\frac{\text{Cash and marketable securities} + \text{long-term investments}}{(\text{Operating expenses} - \text{depreciation}) / 365}$$

for EPFH:

$$\frac{\$38{,}200{,}000 + \$94{,}595{,}000}{(\$327{,}867{,}000 - \$20{,}667{,}000) / 365} = 157.8$$

Cash and marketable securities plus long-term investments are taken from the balance sheet; operating expenses and depreciation are drawn from the revenue/expense summary.

The ratio can be calculated with just cash and marketable securities in the numerator (excluding long-term investments); this is the most conservative measure of liquidity. However, in recent years the marketplace has demanded that health care organizations hold more cash and investments as protection for lenders. Accordingly, the numerator of days of cash on hand portrayed here includes cash and both short-term and long-term investments.

EPFH's days of cash on hand is 157.8 days; the benchmark is 164. An upward trend in this ratio and values above the benchmark are desirable; downward trends and values below the benchmark are undesirable.

Days revenue in accounts receivable ratio focuses on the conversion of what is owed to the organization (accounts receivable) into cash—a critical aspect of financial management and health.

An organization's accounts receivable constantly turn over. Services are provided to patients and accounts receivable increase. Bills are cut and sent to payors or patients. Bills are paid (by patients, health plans, Medicare, Medicaid); one type of current asset (accounts receivable) is decreased and another (cash) is increased. Since accounts receivable are generally a health care organization's largest current asset, how well they are managed is carefully monitored by bond rating agencies and lenders.

This ratio is calculated as:

$$\frac{\text{Net patient accounts receivable}}{\text{Net patient revenue} / 365}$$

for EPFH:

$$\frac{\$67,900,000}{(\$323,100,000 / 365)} = 76.7$$

Net patient accounts receivable is taken from the balance sheet; net patient revenue is drawn from the revenue/expense summary.

EPFH's days in accounts receivable is 76.7 days; it takes about two and one-half months from when a service is provided to the time the account is settled. The benchmark is 66 days. Thus EPFH is taking longer to collect on bills to payors (individuals, governmental programs, and health plans) than peer hospitals; this may indicate it is experiencing problems managing its accounts receivable. Days in accounts receivable affects the amount of cash on hand. Here's an illustration: the average value of one day's worth of revenue for EPFH is about $885,205 (net patient revenues divided by 365). If EPFH reduced its days in accounts receivable by 10 (close to the benchmark), it would produce an additional $9 million ($855,205 times 10) of cash in its "pocket" rather than in the coffers of payors. Additionally, if these funds could be invested at 4 percent interest, annual income would increase by an additional $360,000.

Values of days revenues in accounts receivable below the benchmark and declining trends are desirable; values above the benchmark and increasing trends are undesirable.

Profitability Ratios

Profit provides the means for an organization to develop and grow. Absent an adequate level of profit, the organization must borrow more, its owners (stakeholders, or shareholders) must contribute or invest more, donors must give more, or assets must be sold off (unless they are peripheral, this is an act of cannibalization). Simply put, profits are necessary for an organization to have a future.

Nonprofit Organizations?

The term *nonprofit organization* is the ultimate misnomer. No organization can survive or thrive over the long run without profits—margins generated by an excess of total revenues over total expenses. The amount of profit needed is affected by a host of factors in addition to board and management financial objectives. Even so, ya can't do without it. Thus, nonprofit does not mean *no profit*. Rather, the term describes the way profits are used. In a nonprofit organization, margins cannot be distributed to the inurement of parties outside the organization; this is a requirement of section 501(c)(3) of the Internal Revenue Code. They must remain, and be reinvested, in the organization. Some proportion of the profits of a commercial corporation may be distributed to its owners (stockholders) in the form of dividends, but like nonprofits commercial entities also plow back profits into the business to fuel development and growth.

Total margin is an organization's bottom line, the overall (and the most general) measure of profitability.

$$\frac{\text{Net income}}{\text{Total revenue}}$$

for EPFH:

$$\frac{\$21,748,000}{\$340,700,000} \times 100 = 6.4\%$$

Both net income and total revenue are taken from the revenue/expense summary. The numerator includes net income from all sources, both operating and nonoperating.

Operating margin is calculated as:

$$\frac{\text{Net income from operations}}{\text{Total revenue}}$$

for EPFH:

$$\frac{\$12,833,000}{\$340,700,000} \times 100 = 3.8\%$$

As with total margin, both the numerator and denominator are taken from the revenue/expense summary.

Of total and operating margin ratios, the latter is more important. It reflects profits derived from the organization's core business: providing health care services. EPFH's operating margin is 3.8 percent; a little less than four cents of profit is generated from each dollar of operating revenue. A hospital is typically a thin-margin business; the benchmark is in the neighborhood of 3–4 percent, and many suggest that it should be 5–8 percent. Obviously, upward trends and values above the benchmark range are desirable; the reverse is undesirable.

Roughly 60 percent of EPFH's net income is generated by operations. In health care organizations, most nonoperating income is typically derived from investing activities. Organizations have far more influence over operating margins than over the performance of their financial investments.

Return on equity is the ultimate yardstick of an organization's profitability. In nonprofits this ratio measures how effectively stakeholders' investment (owners equity) is employed to generate profits. It is calculated as:

$$\frac{\text{Net income}}{\text{Owners equity}}$$

for EPFH:

$$\frac{\$21,748,000}{\$250,635,000} \times 100 = 8.7\%$$

Net income is taken from the revenue/expense summary; owners equity comes from the balance sheet.

Recall that owners equity is what an organization is worth—shareholder (in a commercial corporation) or stakeholder (in a nonprofit) initial investment in the business plus reinvested profits. This ratio depicts profits as a percentage of worth.

EPFH was able to generate 8.7 cents of profit for each dollar of equity investment; the benchmark is 5.4 percent. Ratio values exceeding the benchmark and increasing trends are desirable; values below the benchmark and downward trends are undesirable.

Capital Structure Ratios

Capital structure focuses on the right side of the balance sheet and deals with the mix of owner- and lender-supplied funds, the amount of debt an organization has assumed versus owners equity (what it is worth). We return to the topic of capital structure in Chapter Seven.

Debt to equity is a comparison of an organization's total liabilities and the amount of owners equity. It is calculated as:

$$\frac{\text{Total liabilities}}{\text{Owners equity}}$$

for EPFH:

$$\frac{\$117,580,000}{\$250,635,000} \times 100 = 46.9\%$$

Both the numerator and denominator of this ratio are taken from the balance sheet.

EPFH's debt-to-equity ratio is 46.9 percent, meaning the hospital's creditors have lent about 47 cents to the business for every dollar of owners equity in the business. This ratio increases as an organization employs more borrowed funds, or if owners equity decreases because dividends are paid (in commercial corporations), or if losses are experienced.

The ratio is a rough measure of an organization's debt capacity. The benchmark is about 43 percent. This is lower than EPFH's 46.9 percent, indicating that (everything else equal) EPFH may have little capacity to take on additional debt at a reasonable rate of interest.

Lenders like to see lower ratios (fewer liabilities). On the other hand, organizations strive for higher ratios (but not too high), using "other people's money" to fund the business.

Debt service coverage measures an organization's ability to pay back (or service) its debt and is calculated as:

$$\frac{\text{Net income} + \text{depreciation} + \text{interest expense}}{\text{Interest expense} + \text{principal}}$$

for EPFH:

$$\frac{\$21,748,000 + \$20,667,000 + \$3,400,000}{\$3,400,000 + \$3,600,000} = 6.5$$

Net income, depreciation, and interest expense are taken from the revenue/expense summary; principal payments on long-term debt during the current accounting period are taken from the statement of cash flows.

EPFH's debt service coverage ratio is 6.5, which means that it can pay the principal and interest on its debt six and one-half times from the current accounting period's financial performance; the benchmark is 4. EPFH can comfortably pay the principal and interest on its debt. This might indicate that EPFH could borrow more, even though its debt-to-equity ratio exceeds that of peer hospitals. Lenders look at both capacity and coverage when making a decision to extend credit.

Higher debt service coverage ratios and increasing trends are desirable; rates below the benchmark and downward trends are undesirable.

Activity Ratios

Activity ratios indicate how well an organization's different types of assets are being employed to generate revenues (not profits). Assets are resources; they can be deployed effectively or ineffectively to bring revenue into the business.

Total assets turnover is the most general measure of an organization's revenue generating ability. It depicts how effectively all assets are being used to produce revenues; it is calculated as:

$$\frac{\text{Total revenues}}{\text{Total assets}}$$

for EPFH:

$$\frac{\$340,700,000}{\$368,215,000} = .93$$

72

Total revenue is drawn from the revenue/expense summary; total assets is the total of the left side of the balance sheet.

EPFH's ratio is .93, which indicates that each dollar of assets is generating 93 cents of revenue. The benchmark is .97, which says EPFH is generating revenues from its asset base slightly less effectively than peer hospitals. Values of this ratio above the benchmark and an upward trend are desirable; lower values and a downward trend is undesirable.

The denominator can be deflated by old or aging fixed assets (typically the largest piece of total assets), which increases total assets turnover. This brings us to the next activity ratio.

Average age of plant is a measure of the accounting age of an organization's fixed assets. It is calculated as:

$$\frac{\text{Accumulated depreciation}}{\text{Depreciation expense}}$$

for EPFH:

$$\frac{\$208,600,000}{\$20,667,000} = 10.1$$

Accumulated depreciation is shown on the balance sheet; current year depreciation expense is taken from the revenue/expense summary.

EPFH's figure is about 10, and the benchmark is 8.5. Its fixed assets are about one and one-half years older than the standard, indicating that EPFH will likely have to make significant investments in property, plant, and equipment sooner than peer hospitals. Average age of plant is a gross measure but useful in quantifying investment needs. A hospital is a capital-intensive business that experiences rapid technological obsolescence. Attempting to remain competitive with out-of-date facilities and equipment is quite difficult.

Operating Statistics

In addition to basic financial statements, you will likely encounter a summary of operating statistics. Exhibit 6.6 presents an example for EPFH.

Exhibit 6.6. E. Polley Francis Hospital: Illustrative Operating Statistics

	2006	2005	% Change
Admissions	24,500	24,100	1.7%
Patient days	115,000	113,000	1.8%
Average length of stay	4.694	4.689	0.1%
Outpatient visits	310,000	302,000	2.6%
Full-time-equivalent employees (FTE)	2,900	2,850	1.8%
Salaries and benefits per FTE	$54,483	$52,640	3.5%
Case mix index (CMI)	1.066	1.064	0.2%

The number and types of statistics you'll see are more extensive than in this illustration.

The thing to keep in mind is that operations (and the statistics that reflect them) drive finances (and the ratios that portray them). When significant positive or negative changes in financial ratios occur, they warrant an analysis of underlying operations. Your board doesn't need to be concerned with the specifics of interpreting operating statistics and how they affect the organization's financial condition; this is management's job. However, the board should expect management to explain these linkages.

Trends

The previous sections have focused on ratios and statistics for one year or changes between the present and preceding accounting periods. To be really useful, such data must be portrayed as trends; we recommend a minimum of four years. The best, and most board-friendly, way to do so is graphical. Exhibit 6.7 illustrates the key elements.

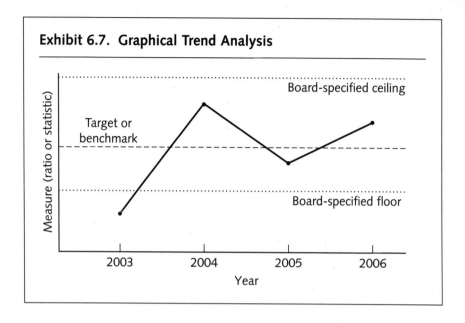

Exhibit 6.7. Graphical Trend Analysis

One measure, ratio, or statistic (vertical axis) is portrayed across the current and past accounting periods (horizontal axis). The graph contains four pieces of information. The solid black line shows actual performance. The dashed line is the benchmark. The two dotted lines are the board-specified ceiling and floor that the measure should not exceed or fall below.

In analyzing ratios and statistics over time, there are four things to look at. The first is the *overall trend and direction.* Is the ratio moving up or down? Is this movement desirable or undesirable (that is, are the ratios or statistics that should be increasing or decreasing doing so)? Second is the *relationship between ratios and statistics.* Ratios and statistics affect one another; look for these connections since they can be important in beginning to understand cause-and-effect relationships; for example, increasing days in accounts receivable decreases days of cash on hand. The third thing to look for is *fluctuation.* Examine ratios and statistics that don't show a definite trend but instead are bouncing up and down. Ask what is causing the fluctuation; what are the implications? Finally, make *comparisons with benchmarks.* Absolute values of ratios and statistics must be compared with benchmarks. An indicator may be moving up or down but be appropriately above or below the benchmark for peer organizations.

FINANCIAL OVERSIGHT

From a governance perspective, the purpose of financial statement analysis is to give a board the means to exercise its oversight role—ensuring that the organization's financial performance meets standards and that its financial condition is healthy and improving.

Key aspects of the financial oversight process are depicted in Exhibit 6.8. The process entails four steps:

1. Select indicators of financial performance and condition (for example, operating margin, days of cash on hand, days in accounts receivable, and debt service coverage).

2. For these indicators, specify standards (a target or benchmark, a range or ceiling above which the measure must not go, a floor below which they shouldn't fall, or some combination of all three).

3. Measure the indicators and compare them with the specified standards.

4. Depending on the results of step three, celebrate and reward accomplishments or else expect an action plan from management to correct the deficiency, and then follow up to ensure the plan is having the desired effect.

To employ the process suggested here and effectively and efficiently oversee a health care organization's financial performance and condition, a board should design and use a "dashboard" system. The dashboard comprises five panels: liquidity, profitability, capital structure, activity, and operating. Each panel has a set of "gauges" (we recommend about a half-dozen) that portray specific financial indicators (ratios or statistics) plus associated standards (acceptable zones, ceilings, floors). The board then employs the dashboard to monitor and oversee organizational financial performance and condition,

Essentials of Health Care Organization Finance

Exhibit 6.8. Board Financial Performance Oversight Process

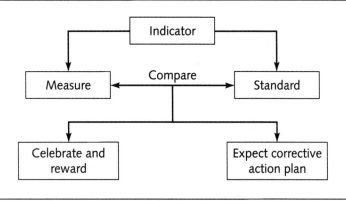

The Frog in Water

Ray Kroc, founder of McDonald's, would often say that if you throw a frog into a pot of boiling water it will jump out. But put a frog in a pot of water and gradually increase the temperature, and it won't jump out; it will boil to death.

The point: the financial performance and condition of many health care organizations is like the frog in the pot of water whose temperature is gradually increasing. The situation progressively gets worse, problems are not addressed, and the board continuously lowers its standards over time until the organization gradually boils to death.

Our admonition: don't get caught in this trap!

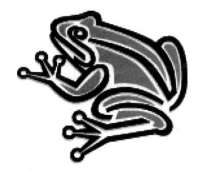

asking questions and expecting corrective actions if all is not going according to plan.

There are two ways to construct a dashboard. In the first approach, the board can specify a set of financial indicators for each panel; there are hundreds from which to choose. The finance committee might develop a long list, from which the board selects specific indicators and standards. In the second *approach,* the board selects a target bond rating that it wants the organization to achieve (say, A or BBB+). Gauges (coupled indicators and standards) are then compiled for that bond rating from benchmark data compiled by rating agencies (Fitch, Moody's Investors Service, Standard & Poor's). Bond ratings are discussed in Chapter Eight.

Either approach can help a board perform its financial oversight role. However, we recommend the second because it is simple, straightforward, and easy to design and use; it constructs the dashboard indicator (gauges) from those that have been validated, and are employed by, rating agencies, bond insurers, investment bankers, and potential lenders.

A board's financial oversight role is to:

- Construct the financial dashboard and specify standards for each gauge or indicator (with input from the CEO and CFO)
- Compare actual performance with standards
- Assess whether the organization is performing in line with expectations
- Address problematic results by ensuring that management develops a plan to correct the deficiencies
- Follow up to make sure the action plan is having the desired effect

A board's job is *not* to formulate operational strategies and tactics to solve problems once they emerge.

IN THE BOARDROOM

➢ Has your board constructed a financial performance/condition dashboard composed of key horizontal and vertical statistics and a comprehensive array of liquidity, profitability, capital structure, activity,

Essentials of Health Care Organization Finance

and operating ratios? Many health care organizations have not implemented this essential oversight tool.

➤ With the heavy lifting done by the finance committee, the financial dashboard should be monitored by your board at least quarterly:

  Which are positive or negative relative to standards and benchmarks? Which are moving in the right or wrong direction? What are the intermediate trends?

  What are the implications for your organization's financial condition in the future?

  If deficiencies are detected, what is management's plan for correcting them?

➤ Make sure your board does not fall into the trap of incrementally adjusting financial targets if performance deteriorates and becoming a "boiled frog" (recall the sidebar). This is why we recommend employing financial indicators that are based on bond rating benchmarks.

➤ Martin Luther King, Jr., was fond of saying, "Keep your eyes on the prize." Good advice for boards. Your role is to set performance standards, monitor financial performance, and expect corrective action from management if all is not going according to plan. It's not your job to come up with solutions to solve problems.

CHAPTER 7

Looking Forward

Vision, Strategies, Financial Plans, and Budgets

OBJECTIVES

After completing this chapter, you will:

- Understand a health care organization's planning cycle, its components, and their interrelationships
- Be familiar with the format, content, preparation, and use of financial plans and budgets
- Be prepared to offer input regarding, and oversee, your organization's financial planning and budgeting process

The preceding three chapters have dealt with basic accounting concepts, financial reporting, and assessing financial performance and condition. The focus has been on an organization's past and present.

In this chapter and the next two we turn to financial planning and decision making that deals with the future, the arena of financial management. This chapter presents an overview of financial planning and budgeting, in addition to vision formulation and strategic planning. Chapter Eight addresses capital structure, creditworthiness, and debt financing. Chapter Nine deals with the use of funds—capital projects and investment decisions.

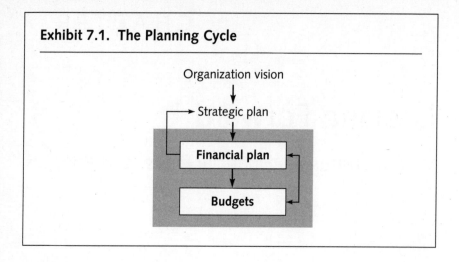

Exhibit 7.1. The Planning Cycle

Organization vision

→ Strategic plan

Financial plan

Budgets

Exhibit 7.1 portrays the financial planning cycle (shaded) in addition to the functions that precede (and create the context for) it. The process is iterative. A strategic plan leads to, and is the basis for, formulating a financial plan. The financial plan is the context for developing budgets. As a result of constantly expressing, analyzing, and testing potential initiatives in financial terms, both financial plans and budgets affect formulation of strategies. This iterative back-and-forth, up-and-down is gone through many times within and across accounting periods.

THE VISION AND STRATEGIC PLANNING

Financial planning and budgeting are grounded in an organization's vision and strategic plan.

A *vision* is a fine-grained image of what an organization should and could become in the future in order to maximize stakeholder benefit. Mention vision and what pops into most people's minds is something like this:

> E. Polley Francis Hospital will become a leader in its market,
> providing the highest-quality care at the lowest possible cost.

This type of generic and vague statement bears no resemblance to the concept of vision that we briefly develop here.

Vision and Mission

A vision focuses on an organization's future, and a mission defines its present; the vision challenges, and the mission anchors. Although both are important, we focus on the vision here. The reason is that an organization can't do anything about where it's at (the mission); but it has considerable influence over where it's headed. Crafting an explicit, precise, coherent, and empowering vision is the critical prerequisite for determining what the organization should become, and then planning (strategically, financially, and operationally) how it should get there.

As illustrated in Exhibit 7.2, a vision is composed of core purposes, core values, and key goals.

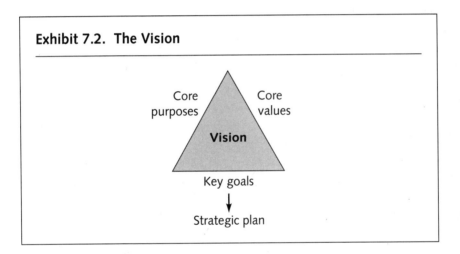

Exhibit 7.2. The Vision

Core purposes are the most important things an organization wants to achieve, answering questions such as these:

- Why should the organization exist, and what should it exist for?
- How should the organization be different from what it is now? What should it strive to become to further stakeholder interests and meet their needs and expectations? How should it remain the same?

- Which markets should the organization serve (and which should it avoid)?
- What types of benefit should be provided to stakeholders, customers, and the community?

Core purposes are an organization's reason for being, in the future.

Core values are the most important ideals an organization embraces as it goes about achieving its purpose, answering such questions as:

- At our very best, what principles guide our planning, decision making, and actions?
- What are the organization's ultimate ethical "thou shalts" and "thou shalt nots"?
- What standards define the organization's heart and soul? What rules should we live by?

Key goals are specific "accomplishables." By formulating them, an organization says to itself, "Above all else, achieve these things." Organization-level goals should be few in number; realistic but stretching; quantifiable, setting targets and clear measures of success or lack thereof; and time-specific, noting when they should be achieved.

Exhibit 7.3 illustrates the core purposes, core values, and key goals for E. Polley Francis Hospital.

Although management and the medical staff provide input to, and participate in, the process, it's a board's responsibility to formulate an organization's vision. It is here where a board exercises the greatest influence over and in an organization on behalf of stakeholders.

An organization's strategic plan (as depicted in Exhibit 7.4) is based on an understanding and analysis of environmental (the economy as a whole and the health care industry) contingencies, constraints, and trends; organizational strengths and weaknesses; and local market opportunities and threats. Strategies are patterns of ideas and actions for deploying an organization's resources to simultaneously gain and sustain advantage vis-à-vis competitors, and offer a high level of value to stakeholders, customers, purchasers, and payors.

Exhibit 7.3. A Vision: E. Polley Francis Hospital, Illustrative Purposes, Values, and Goals

Core purposes

- Focus on providing, in zip codes XXXXX though XXXXX (EPFH's core service area), the full range of health promotion and disease prevention services; primary outpatient services; and primary, secondary, and carefully selected tertiary inpatient services.
- Offering, in association with our partners, health care services perceived by patients, purchasers, and health plans to be in the top quartile in terms of value.
- Providing (at no out-of-pocket cost) the poor, uninsured, and underinsured in our community health care services equal in quality and comprehensiveness available to individuals with standard health insurance coverage.
- Being perceived as an employer of choice in our community; giving our staff opportunities for meaningful work and continuous development at rates of compensation that exceed the norm for comparable positions.
- Remaining a free-standing, independent, nonprofit hospital not affiliated with a system.

Core values

- Respecting the dignity and worth of all persons.
- Maintaining the highest ethical standards in all of our dealings.
- Creating collaborative and mutually empowering relationships with members of our medical staff.
- Being viewed by our community as an exemplary corporate citizen.

Key goals

- Grow weighted outpatient and inpatient market share to 40 percent in our core service area.
- Have 250 physicians in our tightly affiliated medical groups (key partners) by 200X.
- Complete implementation of our comprehensive patient safety program by no later than 200X.
- Be rated in the top 10 percent of our peer group on standardized surveys of clinical quality, patient satisfaction, employee satisfaction, and medical staff satisfaction.

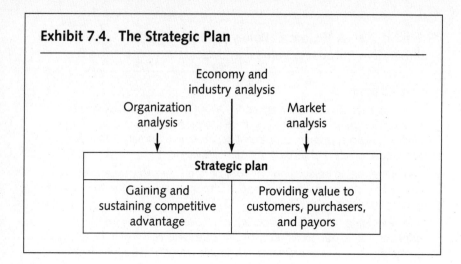

Exhibit 7.4. The Strategic Plan

Economy and
industry analysis

Organization
analysis

Market
analysis

Strategic plan	
Gaining and sustaining competitive advantage	Providing value to customers, purchasers, and payors

Governing and Managing

Governance and management are fundamentally different, but complimentary, functions. Here is the distinction: managing is running the organization, and governing is seeing it's well run. Nowhere is this made clearer than an appropriate and effective subdivision of responsibility for visioning and strategic planning.

To optimize its leverage, the board should focus on understanding stakeholder interests and needs and formulating a vision that leads to maximizing their benefit. The board has the perspective, competence, and wisdom to do these things; indeed, the fundamental obligation of governing (as discussed in Chapter One) demands it. Management should focus on developing strategies, financial plans, and budgets.

Directors and executives have differing vantage points, positions, and roles to play. Directors are in the balcony, orchestrating and overseeing the dance. Executives are on the floor, doing the dancing. Every now and then, directors (especially those who are executives themselves) want to go downstairs and have a dance, or two, or three; it's fun, particularly if they are good at it. They must resist the temptation. The more a board manages, the less it governs.

It is here where the line (albeit a fuzzy one) is drawn between governing and managing (see "Governing and Managing" sidebar): the board envisions the organization and management formulates strategies designed to fulfill that vision. Strategic planning is management's responsibility, but the board should not wash its hands of all things strategic. Here's our recommendation:

- Each year, management develops a set of core strategies accompanied by a concise rationale describing how they are linked with fulfilling the vision.
- The strategies and accompanying rationales are then reviewed by the board. Some questions that might be asked: Are strategies and the vision aligned? Taken as a whole, are strategies coherent, internally consistent, and mutually reinforcing? Are the rationales sound and reasonable?

Strategy execution requires money and necessitates allocating it. Enter financial planning.

FINANCIAL PLANNING

A strategic plan puts forward ideas; the financial plan monetizes them and tests their feasibility, in financial terms, over time.

Financial planning is deciding today what should be done in the future and assessing the financial viability of the decisions. An organization that fails to plan for its future will be overwhelmed and blindsided by it. Recognize that an organization's present and future financial performance and condition, in addition to its capacity to meet community needs, are a direct result of the quality of past financial planning.

Here are some reasons why an organization must do financial planning and have a plan:

- A financial plan analyzes strategies in financial terms, asking: Do they make economic sense? What impact will they have on the organization's future financial performance and condition?
- A financial plan is necessary for execution, linking initiatives developed in the strategic plan with budgets and operational decisions and actions.

- A financial plan assesses the degree of financial risk associated with pursuing various strategies.
- Financial planning is a way to test the impact of a number of scenarios (sets of actions), allowing management to ask a host of *if-then* questions.
- A financial plan is needed to deploy resources effectively.
- A financial plan is a convenient way for management to convey to the board, medical staff, and other leadership groups where the organization is headed and how it will get there.
- Financial planning and plans are required for the organization to have access to capital markets; along with a host of other factors, lenders assess risk on the basis of the quality of an organization's financial planning process and the nature of its plans.

Financial planning and plans are long-range; the question is, how long? The planning time frame (horizon) employed varies with the organization, typically from three to ten years out. We recommend seven years because it often takes this long to plan, execute, and see the initial results of major capital projects (such as building and modernizing facilities).

The problem and challenge of long-range financial planning is that the zone of probable error is a function of time; the number and magnitude of overestimates and underestimates grow as the planning horizon increases. To compensate for (though not eliminate) this problem, organizations can engage in "rolling forward" financial planning. That is, in year zero (the present) the financial plan has a horizon of seven years; at the conclusion of the current accounting period, the financial plan is updated and extended by an additional year, and so on continuously. We recommend this practice.

The financial plan is all about juxtaposing an organization's financial needs with its capacity. Exhibit 7.5 (adapted from *Finance in Brief*, by Kenneth Kaufman) illustrates the relationship between these two critical factors. To be successful and remain viable, an organization must balance financial needs and capacities, irrespective of the magnitude of each. This balance is represented by the line moving from the lower-left corner to the upper-right. At the extremes, low financial capacity is matched with equally low financial needs and great financial needs are accompanied by high financial capacity. Deviation above or below the line entails differing types and amounts of financial risk: relatively low (white), moderate (light gray), and increasingly higher (dark gray).

Needs outstrip capacity with movement along the diagonal arrow in the

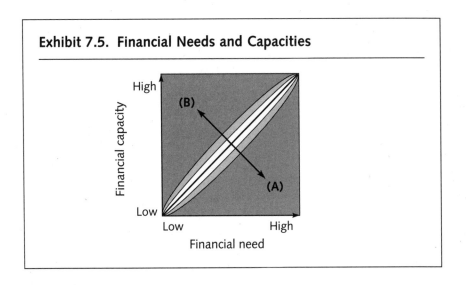

Exhibit 7.5. Financial Needs and Capacities

direction marked A in Exhibit 7.5. Here the organization's financial reach exceeds its grasp. The number or magnitude of strategic ideas cannot be supported by available resources. The risk is overdoing it, spending more funds than the organization has, can borrow, or is able to generate.

Capacity exceeds need and desires with movement along the arrow in the direction marked B; financial reach is less than grasp. Here there is a shortage of strategic ideas or lack of ability or willingness to pursue them. The risk is not effectively deploying available resources for organizational expansion or development in the future.

Simply stated, financial planning and plans align an organization's financial needs and capacity so it can successfully move into the future. This notion is illustrated in Exhibit 7.6. The strategic plan (grounded in an organization's vision) produces financial needs and capacity. Financial needs (uses of funds) include capital investment, working capital, and debt payments. Financial capacity (source of funds) comes from profits, debt, and donations or grants. Financial plans quantify, in dollars, estimates of sources and uses of funds in the future.

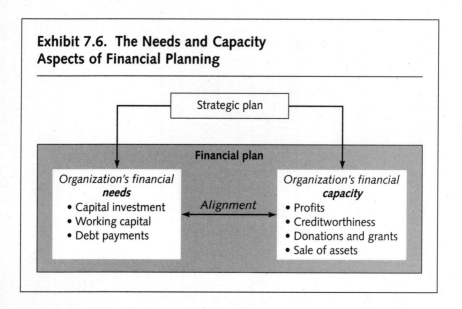

Exhibit 7.6. The Needs and Capacity Aspects of Financial Planning

Strategic plan

Financial plan

Organization's financial **needs**
• Capital investment
• Working capital
• Debt payments

Alignment

Organization's financial **capacity**
• Profits
• Creditworthiness
• Donations and grants
• Sale of assets

Because of the requirements of GAAP, external reporting requirements and custom financial statements look very similar across sectors and organizations. This is not the case with financial plans; their format, content, and (unfortunately) quality and usefulness vary considerably. Accordingly, it's impossible to illustrate a financial plan like the one you may see in your organization and boardroom. However, we can forward an exemplar.

Exhibit 7.7 presents an example of the key components of a financial plan and their relationships. Keep in mind that the plan is based on constant data gathering and analyses. This task has been made easier in recent years because of commercially available computer software; given the large number of linked variables that must be taken into account, sophisticated financial planning would be difficult to do without it.

Essentials of Health Care Organization Finance

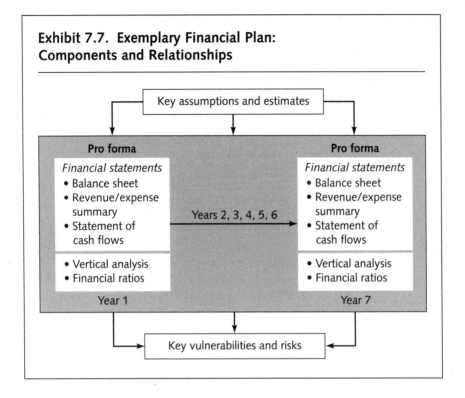

Exhibit 7.7. Exemplary Financial Plan: Components and Relationships

Key assumptions and estimates

Pro forma

Financial statements
- Balance sheet
- Revenue/expense summary
- Statement of cash flows

- Vertical analysis
- Financial ratios

Year 1

Years 2, 3, 4, 5, 6

Pro forma

Financial statements
- Balance sheet
- Revenue/expense summary
- Statement of cash flows

- Vertical analysis
- Financial ratios

Year 7

Key vulnerabilities and risks

Our idealized financial plan has three major components: assumptions and estimates; pro forma (projected) financial statements with associated vertical and ratio analyses; and specification and assessment of vulnerabilities and risks.

First, a financial plan is based on hundreds of assumptions and estimates. They all deal with projected changes across accounting periods, which can have a significant impact on an organization's financial performance and condition in the future. Here are a few illustrations:

- Potential sources and uses of funds—financial capacity and needs
- Board financial policies, such as a target bond rating and associated financial ratios necessary to achieve it
- General economic conditions—in the nation, the industry, and the local market

- Productivity ratios for categories of personnel
- Inflation rate for services and supplies
- Payor mix, regulatory changes, reimbursement rates, and contract terms

Second, these assumptions and estimates are employed to construct projected financial statements and associated analyses for future years. This component of the plan contains pro forma (again, estimated):

- Revenue/expense summaries, balance sheets, and cash flow statements
- Vertical analyses, where the denominators are total revenues for the revenue/expense summaries, total assets for balance sheets, and ending cash balance for statements of cash flows
- Key liquidity, profitability, capital structure, and activity ratios

Third, the financial plan describes and assesses the most important vulnerabilities and risks across accounting periods. Examples of questions addressed include:

- What are the most important things that could go wrong? What is the probability they might happen? What would be their effect on the organization's financial performance and condition?
- What are the most critical capacity constraints that could hinder implementation of the plan (such as the availability of beds or staff resources)?
- How sensitive are key financial ratios to a change in assumption or estimate as reflected in pro forma financial statements?
- What are the most critical success factors?

When all this is brought together in one place, it is the size of the New York City phone book. So, what does a board need to see, and what should be done with it? Under normal circumstances (short of a looming financial crisis), we recommend that (1) important alterations in components of the financial plan (assumptions, estimates, pro forma financial statements and analyses, and vulnerabilities and risks) be presented to, and reviewed by, the finance committee twice a year; and (2) a summary of the financial plan (based on finance committee review) should be presented to, and discussed by, the full board annually. There is some debate about whether a board should formally approve the financial plan. We recommend doing so, with the proviso that what's being approved is management's plan, not the board's; that is, management owns the plan, and the board ratifies it.

BUDGETING

A budget is a detailed management planning and control tool that describes how resources will be obtained and deployed in the present and near-term accounting periods. The typical health care organization develops a budget for the organization as a whole (in addition to ones for major operating components, which will not be addressed here). The financial plan sets the context for preparing budgets; the budgets lay out all the detail required to formulate a financial plan. Again we see an iterative cycle of activity.

Directors need a general feel of what budgets are, the various ways they can be developed, and how they can be employed as monitoring and control tools.

There are five components of an organization-wide budget: statistical, revenue, expense, capital, and cash. They are linked together and must be constructed in tandem. Budgets are prepared for the forthcoming accounting period.

The *statistical* budget component is the foundation for (and it drives) the revenue/expense components. It projects the volume of specific services to be provided. Illustrative volume projections include admissions, patient days, outpatient and emergency room visits, number of covered lives, and case mix. The statistical budget component is important because it ensures that all others are based on the same set of volume estimates.

The *revenue* budget component takes estimated volumes for specific services and multiplies them by expected payments, given the organization's payor and service mix. This is an exceedingly complex process, due to differing reimbursement rates and contract terms and changes in them. Additionally, deductions from revenue (such as discounts and uncompensated care) must be figured in.

The *expense* budget component estimates the cost of providing the volume of services projected in the statistics budget as reflected in the revenue budget. It's summarized in four expense types: personnel, supplies, and capital, plus the catch-all of "other." Personnel expenses (the big-ticket item because health care organizations are so labor-intensive) incorporate staffing mix, number of employees by category, wage rates, and productivity ratios. Supplies include estimates of the type and amount that will be used and price per unit. Capital costs include depreciation and interest expenses.

The *capital* budget component estimates the cost of acquiring the fixed assets needed to generate projected levels of service volume. Major categories include buying property, building and modernizing facilities, replacing equipment, and acquiring new technology.

The *cash* budget component projects cash inflows and outflows and their timing, plus estimating the sources and uses of cash.

In addition to being critical for financial planning, budgets are also employed to monitor and control. The tool for doing so is *variance analysis*—presentation and evaluation of differences between what was budgeted and actual results. Look at the budget and its various components as promises made by management. The board must compare these promises with results. If there are significant variances, either plus or minus, understand the reason; if problems are detected, expect management to have a plan to correct them.

With regard to board involvement in the budgeting process, we recommend that:

- The budget should be presented to, but not be approved by, the finance committee or the full board (unless required by law, as is the case with many governmental health care organizations)
- Organization-wide statistics, revenue, expense, capital, and cash budget components be reviewed by the finance committee
- Summaries of major budget variances be presented to and discussed by the board twice each year

IN THE BOARDROOM

➤ Review the vision. It should be a precise, explicit, fine-grained, coherent, and empowering specification of what your organization will become in the future to maximize stakeholder benefit. It should also be a product of your board's effort and deliberation (with input from management and the medical staff). Visioning requires making important and difficult choices (the organization should head this way and accomplish these things). Formulating a vision is the most important way your board exercises influence over and in the organization. If your board's visioning does not pass muster regarding either process or substance, then doing some serious work here is good use of a retreat.

➤ Annually, management should present to your board and flesh out its key strategies. Each strategy should be explicitly linked to the vision. The question that must be asked by your board is, How does pursuing this particular strategy contribute to fulfilling the vision and enhancing stakeholder value?

➤ How is financial planning done in your organization?

Is there a succinct and focused financial plan that contains key assumptions and estimates, pro forma financial statements (revenue/expense summaries, balance sheets, and statements of cash flows) plus vertical and ratio analyses, and an assessment of key vulnerabilities and risks?

Does your board revisit financial plans for past accounting periods and assess how things actually worked out? Your board must continuously evaluate whether, and to what extent, plans have been achieved.

➤ Your board (with governance staff work done by the finance committee) should talk through management's key assumptions and estimates underlying the financial plan. Focus your attention on changes in service volumes, market share (overall and by major service lines), costs (driven by both inflation and utilization), labor productivity, and new debt. Here are key questions your board should ask: How were the estimates developed? How accurate have estimates been in the past? What are the major vulnerabilities if estimates prove to be wrong?

➢ The organization's strategic plan, financial plan, and budget must be linked; changes in one affect the other two. Additionally, your board should expect these linkages will be explicitly articulated by management.

CHAPTER 8

Source of Funds

Financing

OBJECTIVES

After completing this chapter, you will understand:

- Your organization's capital structure—the relative proportion of debt and equity employed to fund the business in addition to the financial risks associated with different mixes

- The importance of creditworthiness and factors affecting it

- Long-term debt financing and key features of bonds and the issuing process

Money is the fuel of business, in for-profits and nonprofits alike. Having enough of it at the right time is critical to a health care organization's success and its ability to provide necessary services. This chapter focuses on sources of financing, with an emphasis on debt.

Most of us couldn't function without incurring some debt, such as automobile loans and home mortgages. The same is true of organizations; they use debt for some part of their financial "fuel supply." Accordingly, a health care organization board must understand and be able to address issues regarding capital structure, creditworthiness, and long-term debt financing.

CAPITAL STRUCTURE

There are two sources of funds available to finance an organization's capital investment needs: equity and debt. Equity financing comes from stakeholder contributions, donations and grants, and retained earnings. Debt financing is provided by lenders and creditors and can be short-term or long-term. Short-term debt is incurred for less than one year and takes a variety of forms, among them extension of credit by vendors and bank loans; it is treated as a current liability on the balance sheet. Long-term debt is typically used to finance major investments in property, plant, equipment, and programs; it is raised through sale of bonds, assuming mortgages, and entering into capital leases.

Both equity and debt serve the same purpose: to produce the financing necessary to run, develop, and expand the business. In 2003 the typical non-profit hospital employed about 5 percent short-term debt, 33 percent long-term debt, and 62 percent equity financing.

Recall from Chapter Five the accounting equation:

$$\text{Assets} = \text{Liabilities} + \text{Owners equity}$$

That is, an organization's assets (what it owns) are financed by a combination of liabilities (some form of debt) and owners equity (what it's worth).

Capital structure deals with composition of the right-hand side of an organization's balance sheet. How "heavy" is the top (liabilities) section of the right side of the balance sheet compared to the bottom (owners equity)? The relative balance between debt and equity is referred to as "leverage"; a business that uses considerably more debt than is typical for its industry is said to be highly leveraged.

An organization's capital structure can be quantified by its debt-to-equity ratio (introduced in Chapter Six):

$$\frac{\text{Total liabilities}}{\text{Owners equity}}$$

For EPFH it is .47, meaning the hospital is financed with 47 cents of debt for every dollar of owners equity. There are (theoretically) an infinite number of capital structure options, ranging from 100 percent equity financing, through a 50-50 split, to 100 percent debt financing.

Executives and boards must determine the mix of debt and equity that will be employed.

- As an organization increases its use of debt, lender risk increases (everything else equal, greater debt service increases the possibility of default). As a consequence, lenders will demand higher interest rates, which increases an organization's cost of capital (and its operating expenses).
- Similarly, as the amount of equity financing decreases and debt increases, an organization has greater leverage (the benefits of using other people's money to finance the business). Again, everything else equal, certain financial performance measures (such as return on equity) improve and stakeholder risks decrease.

Leverage: An Illustration

An organization's net income is $100,000 and its total liabilities plus owners equity (right-hand side of the balance sheet) is $1 million. Here is the impact of two capital structures on the financial ratio return on equity:

$$\frac{\text{Net income}}{\text{Owners equity}} \times 100 = \text{Return on equity}$$

If owners equity is $1,000,000 and debt is zero, then return on equity is 10 percent:

$$\frac{\$100,000}{\$1,000,000} \times 100 = 10\%$$

If liabilities plus owners equity are still $1 million but the business is financed with 50 percent debt ($500,000) and 50 percent owners equity ($500,000), return on equity is 20 percent:

$$\frac{\$100,000}{\$500,000} \times 100 = 20\%$$

The relative amount of equity and debt financing employed depends upon the organization's capital requirements, determined by its strategic and financial plans as addressed in Chapter Seven; and how much additional debt the organization can assume given its creditworthiness.

CREDITWORTHINESS

Creditworthiness is a measure of lenders' collective willingness to extend additional debt financing to an organization. Here's the catch-22: creditworthiness influences an organization's access to capital, which in turn affects its financial condition; but financial condition ultimately determines creditworthiness. These relationships underpin the often-made observation that it's easiest to borrow money when you don't need it (because of your financial health).

There are a number of benefits that flow to an organization from better creditworthiness:

- Lower interest rates when assuming additional debt such as issuing bonds
- Greater access to credit enhancement (bond insurance) at more favorable rates
- Less restrictive lender requirements (bond covenants)
- Access to the taxable (in addition to tax-exempt) debt market
- Less of a requirement to set aside reserve funds to cover debt service payments
- Increased attractiveness of the organization to potential partners (joint ventures, affiliations, mergers, and acquisitions)

Creditworthiness is reflected by a bond rating, which is a judgment regarding an organization's ability to make full and timely interest and principal payments. Rating agencies assess an organization's creditworthiness at the time bonds are issued and periodically thereafter. The initial rating influences the interest rate (and other costs) that an organization will pay for the loan. Subsequent ratings affect bond values in secondary markets (transactions among sellers and buyers of bonds).

Categories and specific ratings employed by the largest bond rating agencies (FitchRatings, Moody's Investors Service, and Standard and Poor's) are depicted in Exhibit 8.1. Using the most fine-grained scale (Fitch) as an illustration, the ratings are interpreted as follows:

AAA	Highest credit quality; the lowest expectation of credit risk, reflecting exceptional capacity for full and timely payment of debt service and retirement of principal
AA	Very high credit quality
A	High credit quality
BBB	Good credit quality; moderate expectation of credit risk
BB	Speculative; possibility of credit risk
B	Highly speculative
CCC, CC, C	High possibility of default (ordered by increasing risk)
DDD, DD, D	In default

Exhibit 8.1. Bond Rating Categories and Scales

Fitch	Moody's	Standard & Poor's
AAA	Aaa	AAA
AA	Aa	AA
A	A	A
BBB	Baa	BBB
BB	Ba	BB
B	B	B
CCC	Caa	CCC
CC	caa	CC
C		
DDD	Ca	D
DD	C	
D		

Bonds rated in the top (dark-shaded) category are investment grade. Most bonds are bought, in both primary and secondary markets, by institutional investors (such as mutual funds, pension funds, and insurance companies); they are often restricted to purchasing issues rated BBB or higher. The middle (light-shaded) category ratings are called "junk bonds"—below investment grade, but not presently in default. The bottom (dark-shaded) bonds are in default; they reflect rating agency estimates of the probability that an organization will be able to make full repayment of principal after reorganization or through liquidation.

Bond ratings are affected by general factors: condition of the economy as a whole, and of the sector or industry in which the organization operates (for example, communications, utilities, health care); and type of organization (for example, health system, hospital, nursing home, multispecialty group practice, HMO, and so on). In addition to general factors, which affect all businesses or those in a particular industry category, the strength of the organization issuing the bond is evaluated. Here are some dimensions (and illustrative components) employed:

- *Nature of the market*—size and rate of growth; social, demographic, and economic characteristics; whether the organization is positioned in one market or several; the organization's market share and whether it is a dominator or leader in its market(s); intensity and volatility of competition
- *Corporate structure* (for health systems)—number and type of subsidiaries and legal relationships among them; composition of the obligated group (borrowing organizations); degree of integration (strategic, financial, operational, and clinical)
- *Governance*—experience, competencies, and involvement of directors; nature of infrastructure in place (bylaws, principles, protocols); mix of outside and inside directors; structure, membership, and functioning of committees (particularly finance and audit)
- *Management*—demonstrated competence, education and experience, longevity
- *Program and service array*—comprehensiveness and breadth of offerings; market leadership and profitability of service lines; teaching affiliation

- *Medical staff*—organization (as reflected in the medical staff's bylaws); quality (proportion of staff that is board-certified and eligible); average age and specialty mix; dependence (percentage of admissions generated by top 20 percent of admitters); tightness of affiliation; nature of relationships with large single-specialty and multispecialty medical groups
- *Nursing*—mix (RNs and LVNs, and by type of training, such as M.N., B.S.N., A.A., and diploma); turnover rate and percentage of vacant positions; retention rate and average longevity of employment; staff satisfaction (as measured by standardized questionnaires); unionization and labor relations history

Since a bond rating reflects an organization's estimated ability to make timely interest and principal payments, the organization-specific factor most affecting creditworthiness is financial performance and condition. Rating agencies undertake a comprehensive and detailed analysis of an organization's audited and projected financial statements; particular attention is paid to capital structure and liquidity ratios.

Exhibit 8.2 presents bond rating financial ratios, and Exhibit 8.3 shows bond rating distributions.

LONG-TERM DEBT FINANCING

Most health care organization long-term debt is financed through the sale of bonds. A bond is a contract (typically twenty to thirty years in duration) registered with the Securities and Exchange Commission that is offered to individuals and institutions, where the borrower agrees to make periodic payments of interest to lenders and repay the principal at maturity.

Entering the capital market and issuing bonds is an important event and obligation entailing significant work and cost, with much at stake. Here is a brief rundown of the key parties typically involved in a bond financing:

- *Borrower.* This is the recipient of funds generated by the bond issue, the entity ultimately responsible for payment of interest and principal. This can be an individual organization or a collection of them (called an obligated group).

Exhibit 8.2. Bond Ratings: Selected Financial Ratios (U.S. Nonprofit Health Systems and Hospitals, 2003)

Measure	Medians by Rating			
	AA	A	BBB	Below BBB
Days of cash on hand	194	155	112	40
Days in accounts receivable	58	57	56	59
Cushion ratio	17	11	6	3
Days in current liabilities	67	62	64	82
Cash to debt (%)	120	100	66	28
Operating margin (%)	2.8	1.8	0.7	–3.0
Excess margin (%)	3.0	2.9	1.4	–1.6
Cash flow from operations before interest margin (%)	10.8	10.7	8.6	7.2
Bad debt expense as a % of total operating revenue	4.4	5.2	5.2	5.5
Maximum annual debt service as a % of total revenues	3.1	3.5	3.5	4.7
Debt to capitalization (%)	36	39	49	79
Debt to assets (%)	29	31	36	46
Average age of plant (years)	9.4	9.2	9.1	12.1
Capital expenditures as a % of depreciation expenses	144	152	125	64

Source: Health Care Special Report, "2003 Median Ratings for Nonprofit Hospitals and Health Care Systems," FitchRatings, www.fitchratings.com.

Exhibit 8.3. Distribution of Bond Ratings (U.S. Nonprofit Health Systems and Hospitals, 2003)

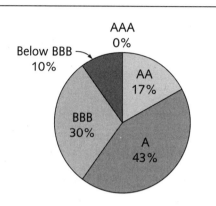

Source: Health Care Special Report, "2003 Median Ratings for Nonprofit Hospitals and Health Care Systems," FitchRatings, www.fitchratings.com.

- *Issuing authority.* This entity is involved in the transaction when bonds are issued by a governmental agency (state, municipality, or district) on behalf of the borrower in order to gain tax-exempt status.
- *Investment banker.* An investment banking firm may play two roles. First, it can act as an advisor to the borrowing organization regarding the structure of the financing, setting interest rates and coordinating activities of parties involved in the transaction and the process of issuing bonds. Second, it can serve as a broker or intermediary between the borrower and the market, responsible for the sale of bonds. There are two types of broker relationship: *best effort,* in which the investment banker puts forward its best effort to sell the bonds, but those unsold remain the property of the borrowing organization; and *underwriter,* wherein the investment banking institution buys some or all of the issue (at a discount) and is at risk for their sale.
- *Market.* This comprises the individual and institutional investors who might purchase the bonds to obtain a return on their investment. They are

willing to assume risk and forgo alternative use of their funds for a specified rate of interest over a period of time.

- *Trustee.* A trustee is typically a commercial bank that serves as a fiscal intermediary and agent of lenders once bonds are sold. The trustee receives proceeds from the sale and delivers funds to the borrowing organization, collects debt service payments from the borrower and distributes interest and principal payments to bond holders, and exercises the terms of the bond indenture (a legal contract) on behalf of lenders.
- *Bond insurer.* If credit enhancement is employed, this insuring company guarantees the lender will receive promised interest and principal payments should the borrower be unable to make them.
- *Feasibility consultant.* Typically, this is a certified public accounting firm or a consulting firm with financial expertise that assesses the organization's financial projections and estimates its ability to service the debt.
- *Legal counsel.* This is a firm retained to identify, address, and resolve the myriad legal issues (including tax exemption) associated with financing, drafting, and reviewing bond indenture documents on behalf of the borrower.

The types and provisions of individual bond issues vary considerably with the needs and creditworthiness of the borrower, in addition to the market status at the time of issue.

The major *types of bonds* include:

- *Debenture.* Any form of unsecured bond. Assurance of debt service and repayment of principal is based on the good faith, creditworthiness, and underlying financial strength of the borrower.
- *Mortgage bond.* The borrower pledges specific real property as collateral for repayment of debt. If the organization defaults on the bonds, the property is claimed by the trustee bank and sold to satisfy obligations to lenders.
- *Municipal bond* (called a "muni" or tax-exempt). An obligation issued by a governmental entity on behalf of a borrowing organization. Although

Essentials of Health Care Organization Finance

there may be restrictions, the interest received by lenders is exempt from federal and many states' income taxes. Because of this, they carry a lower interest rate than taxable issues of similar risk. Most states have authorities that allow nonprofit health care organizations to issue tax-exempt bonds through them.

- *Taxable bond.* A bond issued by the borrowing organization directly, not a governmental entity on its behalf. These bonds are frequently used to finance projects that are not tax-exempt. The interest received by lenders is subject to ordinary federal and state income taxes.

- *Placement.* Bonds can be either sold publicly (to all comers in the market) or privately placed. In the latter arrangement, the issue is sold to one, or a very few, investors (typically large institutions such as pension or mutual funds) through direct negotiation.

Irrespective of type and method of placement, bonds have different *features.* Here are brief descriptions of common provisions:

- *Interest (coupon) rate.* This is the rate a borrower pays lenders for use of their money. Interest on bonds is paid quarterly or semiannually; principal is generally returned to lenders at the bond's maturity date.
- *Call provisions.* These give borrowers the right to pay off all (or a portion of) a bond issue before the maturity date, typically for a premium payment. When this provision is in place, a borrower may call the bonds if interest rates decline significantly; old debt is replaced by newer debt at a lower rate.
- *Credit enhancement.* The most common form of credit enhancement is bond insurance, a mechanism for guaranteeing the lender will receive full and timely payments of interest and principal. It provides protection to lenders against borrower default. In purchasing credit enhancement, the borrower replaces its bond rating with that of the insurer (typically AAA), thus lowering the issue's interest rate. Bond insurance comes at a price, typically stated in terms of basis points (100 points equals one percent). The rate is affected by the borrower's creditworthiness and market conditions.

- *Covenants.* Conditions and restrictions may be required of the borrowing organization by lenders in the bond indenture (contract). A typical covenant provision is specification of financial ratio values that must be maintained by the organization through the bond's maturity; if these values are not maintained, the trustee on behalf of lenders may take actions spelled out in the bond indenture (such as forcing immediate payment of the outstanding principal). Another covenant is a condition that must be satisfied for the organization to issue additional debt.

- *Retirement schedule.* Typically, bonds are retired and principal is returned to lenders at maturity. In some instances the bond indenture provides for sequenced retirement; that is, a percentage of the issue is redeemed according to a specific phased schedule.

- *Reserve fund.* This requires the borrowing organization to place a specified number of years of debt service payments in a restricted fund held by the trustee. In instances where the creditworthiness of the borrower is problematic, this affords an additional level of protection for lenders.

IN THE BOARDROOM

➤ If your organization has done a bond financing in the last several years, request a copy of the bond document from management and look it over. It's a great source of information about the industry, local market, organizational strengths and weaknesses, and the organization's financial performance and condition as well as creditworthiness.

➤ What are your organization's present capital structure and its debt-to-equity ratio? What has been the trend of this ratio over the last five years?

➤ How many bond issues are in place? What are the range of interest rates and weighted average rate across all issues? Much of this information can be found in footnotes to the audited financial statements.

➤ If your organization has outstanding bond issues, does the finance committee and the full board receive periodic reports from management on performance vis-à-vis covenants? Has your organization ever been in violation of a bond covenant (so called technical default)?

➤ Does your organization have bond issues where it has been required to establish a reserve fund? Why were reserves required? (Note that this is not an unusual requirement and does not, in and of itself, signify a financial problem.)

➤ What is your organization's bond rating? How has the rating changed over the last five years? What has been the nature of upgrades and downgrades? What is management's explanation for them?

➤ How do ratios in your organization's financial plan (Chapter Seven) compare with credit rating agency ratios such as those presented in Exhibit 8.2?

➤ At least annually, on the basis of preparatory work undertaken by the finance committee, does your board review the organization's creditworthiness and management's plan to maintain or improve it? We strongly recommend this governance practice.

➤ Is your organization contemplating a bond financing in the next five years? How much? Has this been discussed by your board's finance committee in conjunction with its review of the financial plan?

➤ Who is your organization's investment banker? Does your organization work with the firm continuously or just when a bond issue is being contemplated? If management meets periodically with the investment banker, does your board finance committee review and discuss reports regarding the organization's capital structure, creditworthiness, bond rating, debt capacity, and changes in debt market expectations?

CHAPTER 9

Use of Funds

Capital Investment

OBJECTIVES

After completing this chapter, you will understand:

- The importance of capital investment decisions
- Approaches that have been used by health care organizations to assess proposed capital investments
- How payback and net present value techniques can be employed to analyze the financial worthiness of capital projects
- Your board's role in the capital allocation process

This chapter deals with major capital investment decisions; part of the processes covered in the previous two chapters and depicted in Exhibit 9.1. The question is, How should an organization use resources obtained through the financing process (addressed in Chapter Eight) to make investments designed to accomplish its strategic and financial plans (covered in Chapter Seven)?

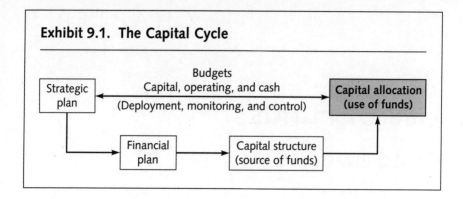

Exhibit 9.1. The Capital Cycle

Strategic plan

Budgets
Capital, operating, and cash
(Deployment, monitoring, and control)

Capital allocation
(use of funds)

Financial plan

Capital structure
(source of funds)

Allocation of capital is among a health care organization's most important decisions because it:

- Defines an organization and affects its future—what it is, the benefits it provides, the extent it's able to fulfill the vision on behalf of the community and stakeholders, its ability to attract medical staff (and ultimately patients), and its competitiveness in the market
  - Has a significant effect on financial and operational performance
  - Entails the commitment of significant resources over time
  - Is often difficult and costly to reverse; once funds are committed to one project rather than another, it's hard to get them back or significantly change direction
- Influences an organization's ability to generate and acquire capital in the future

Accordingly, a board must formulate policies regarding, make decisions about, and oversee an organization's capital allocation process:

- On the basis of strategic and financial plans, ensuring that an appropriate amount of funds are generated and set aside to meet the organization's long-term capital investment needs

Essentials of Health Care Organization Finance

- Making sure management has a capital investment evaluation system in place that

  Considers all nonemergency projects annually, at one point in time

  Combines like-type projects into categories on the basis of explicit criteria (such as risk and the amount of funding requested)

  Subjects all projects in a particular category to the same evaluation and approval process

  Employs appropriate and standardized methods and techniques to analyze the financial attractiveness of projects

  Supplements financial assessment with other important criteria (such as the extent to which a project is aligned with the vision and increases competitive advantage)

- Approving specific capital projects that are of a magnitude and importance warranting the board's attention
- Assessing the effectiveness and efficiency of the capital allocation process; that is, looking back and comparing actual performance of investments to what was anticipated in the proposal

APPROACHES

There are many ways to make capital investment decisions, not all of which are equally good. Some of the more common approaches, often employed in combination, are:

- *Popularity.* Decisions to fund projects are made on the basis of their general attractiveness and appeal, subjectively defined. Each proposal is assessed on a first-come, first-served basis using various criteria in nonstandardized ways.
- *Historical.* Capital is allocated according to past practice; that is, a division's percentage of the "capital pie" in previous years is the baseline for

determining future allocations. The underlying rational is to stay with what has worked in the past.

- *Political.* "Pet projects" of individuals and groups with the most influence receive the greatest attention and have the highest probability of being undertaken. Approval of projects depends on the power of proposers.

- *Championship.* Projects with the most vocal, persistent, and articulate sponsors tend to be funded; those with less support receive little or no attention. The notion is that, lacking a dedicated champion, a project will fail; it's best to bet on the jockey, not just the horse.

- *Mimic.* Capital is deployed in roughly the same way as in similar organizations. Since it's difficult to quantify the attractiveness of different projects, the safest and most prudent course is to do the same as others are doing. The rush of hospitals to purchase physician practices in the 1990s is an illustration of this approach.

These approaches were often satisfactory through the late 1980s in an industry characterized by generous capital markets, minimal competition, and reimbursement that was based on incurred costs or billed charges—all of which buffered health care organizations from capital allocation missteps and mistakes.

The situation has changed: capital is scarce, competition has increased, and reimbursement is far less generous. Altered circumstances warrant different approaches. Popularity, historical, political, championship, and mimic factors will always influence capital investment decisions (and probably should, to some degree), but a more rational and objective process of accessing and approving projects is warranted. Furthermore, it's the board's responsibility to ensure that such a process is in place.

TYPES OF CAPITAL INVESTMENT

A health care organization has a variety of capital investment needs that pose different challenges for making decisions regarding whether they should be pursued. Illustrative categories of capital projects include mandates, operational improvements, expansion, offering line extensions, large building projects, and major new initiatives.

Mandated capital projects are required by law, court decisions, regulations, or accreditation requirements. Accordingly, an organization has little discretion whether to undertake them (although it retains considerable control regarding the "how"). Examples are the need to replace a boiler because of a safety code violation, upgrade a facility's disability access to comply with federal regulations, undertake a building retrofit because of new state earthquake safety standards, and improve a clinical information system to meet accreditation requirements.

Operating improvements are projects intended to enhance the effectiveness or efficiency of how things are presently done in the organization. Many can be big-ticket items requiring major investment, such as the need to install an electronic physician order entry and medical record system, purchase the next generation of diagnostic imaging technology, and modernize existing facilities.

Expansion of existing programs and facilities occurs when capacity exists, but it's inadequate—for example, increasing the number of operating rooms.

Offering line extensions adds new programs. These investments build on, and expand, an organization's present array or mix of services (such as developing a women's health or outpatient surgery program).

Major building encompasses large replacement and capacity expansion projects such as adding a floor or wing to an existing building, remodeling a facility, and new construction.

Major new initiatives are undertaken when an organization enters markets in which it has no previous presence or experience. For a short-term general hospital, this might be developing a health insurance plan, purchasing physician practices, or buying a nursing home.

There are, of course, many ways to categorize capital investment projects, and they are rarely mutually exclusive. However, an organization must have some scheme in place to do so. The reason why is illustrated in Exhibit 9.2; risk varies by project type and size.

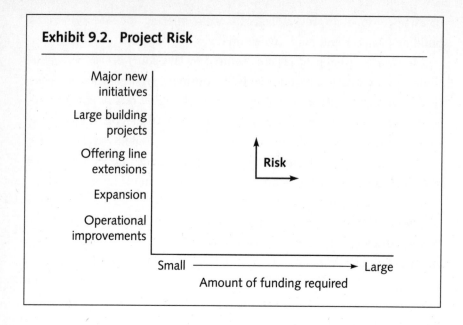

Exhibit 9.2. Project Risk

Major new initiatives

Large building projects

Offering line extensions

Expansion

Operational improvements

Risk

Small ——————→ Large

Amount of funding required

- The risk associated with mandated capital investments is irrelevant. The organization has no choice; they must be undertaken.
- Other types of capital investment are noted on the vertical dimension in terms of increasing risk. For example, everything else equal, operational improvements (incremental changes) are less risky than major new initiatives (doing something totally different).
- The horizontal dimension focuses on the magnitude of capital investment required. Risk varies with the amount of resources that must be committed.

Projects with varying degrees of risk should be subjected to different evaluation and approval processes. For example, low-risk projects (such as operational improvements requiring small expenditures) might be assessed through a quick and simple process and authorized by department heads. Very-high-risk projects (such as a construction program necessitating large investments committed for a long period of time) would move through a much more stringent process and require board-level approval. We recommend that explicit criteria be developed by management (then reviewed

Essentials of Health Care Organization Finance

and approved by the board), specifying the process that will be employed to assess and authorize capital projects of differing risks.

We turn now to the type of rigorous and thorough process that should be employed to make significant capital investment decisions that replace (or complement) the approaches described previously. These processes have been used in other industries for decades and are only now being adopted in health care.

FINANCIAL ANALYSIS OF CAPITAL PROJECTS

Financial analysis of a proposed capital project addresses a number of questions:

- What amount of up-front investment is required to initiate the project?
- How much net cash will the project generate over its life?
- What is the relative payback or return that can be expected from the project when compared with alternative uses of funds?

Analytical Factors

Factors employed to analyze the financial attractiveness of proposed capital projects are depicted in Exhibit 9.3.

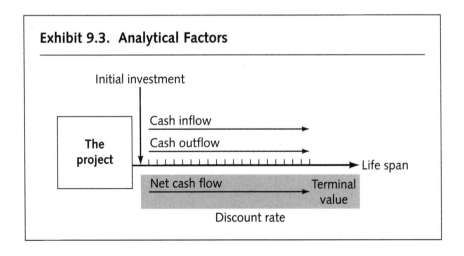

Exhibit 9.3. Analytical Factors

- *The project.* In the past, capital investments were defined narrowly—typically, only large equipment purchases and construction activities. A more contemporary (and, we believe, appropriate) definition is any organizational initiative designed to produce long-term benefits that requires allocation of significant resources. This would include (in addition to property, plant, and equipment) investments in new programs, and service enhancements.
- *Project life span.* The number of years a project will exist.
- *Initial investment.* The up-front investment that must be committed to launch a project includes, for example: the costs of new property, facilities, and equipment; facilities modification; and consulting and legal fees. Such investments must be incremental, attributable directly to the project, and not incurred in the past. For example, if a project uses an existing facility that must be modified, renovation costs would be included, whereas the past expenditure to build it would not.
- *Net cash flow.* The amount of net cash (inflows minus outflows), by accounting period, that a project is estimated to generate over its life span.
- *Terminal value.* Net cash flow that is estimated to be generated in years beyond the project life span. This recognizes that the analytical time frame is often somewhat arbitrary and the project may produce cash flows beyond this point.
- *Discount rate.* This is an estimate of the organization's cost of capital used to discount (adjust) the value of future cash flows generated by the project into present dollars.

Employing these factors, Exhibit 9.4 presents an illustration of cash flow calculations for a proposed capital project with a life span of five years. Several estimates are made:

- Up-front outlays required to start the project (referred to as time zero); this includes an initial capital investment of $2.5 million and associated costs of $735,000, for a total net negative cash flow at time zero of $3,235,000
- Operating cash inflows and outflows for five accounting periods over the project's life span

Exhibit 9.4. Illustrative Cash Flows: Proposed Capital Project

	Year 0	Year 1	Year 2	Year 3	Year 4	Year 5
Initial capital investment	-$2,500,000					
Associated costs	-$735,000					
Gross revenues		$835,000	$1,265,000	$1,456,000	$1,732,000	$2,123,000
Deductions		-$183,500	-$278,000	-$315,000	-$375,000	-$460,000
Cash in =		*$651,500*	*$987,000*	*$1,141,000*	*$1,357,000*	*$1,663,000*
Labor costs		-$62,500	-$78,900	-$83,400	-$92,400	-$98,700
Supplies		-$44,500	-$47,000	-$48,400	-$51,200	-$53,400
Incremental overhead		-$13,200	-$14,100	-$14,600	-$15,800	-$16,100
Other		-$6,100	-$6,800	-$7,100	-$7,300	-$7,800
Cash out =		*-$126,300*	*-$146,800*	*-$153,500*	*-$166,700*	*-$176,000*
Net operating cash flow =		$525,200	$840,200	$987,500	$1,190,300	$1,487,000
Terminal cash flow						$480,900
Net cash flow =	-$3,235,000	$525,200	$840,200	$987,500	$1,190,300	$1,967,900
Cumulative net cash flows =	-$3,235,000	-$2,709,800	-$1,869,600	-$882,100	$308,200	$2,276,100

- Net operating cash flows (cash in minus cash out) for each accounting period
- Cumulative net cash flows, added across accounting periods and including any estimated cash flows beyond year five (the project's terminal value)

Using this information, one can employ several techniques to analyze a proposed capital investment. Two of the most widely used and best—payback and net present value analysis—are described here.

Payback Analysis

Payback period quantifies the time to project break-even, that is, when cumulative net cash flow covers the initial investment.

The information needed to conduct the analysis (drawn from Exhibit 9.4) is depicted in Exhibit 9.5. Cumulative net cash flow turns from negative (−$882,100) to positive ($308,200) in year four. The question is, When? The answer is found by dividing the cumulative net cash flow in the last negative year by the annual cash flow in the first positive year:

$$\frac{\text{Cumulative net cash flow year 3}}{\text{Annual cash flow in year 4}}$$

$$\frac{\$882,100}{\$1,190,300} = .74$$

Time to breakeven is .74 years into the fourth year; payback occurs at about three years and nine months.

The fewer years to payback, the sooner funds invested in a project begin to generate a positive cash flow that can then be used for other purposes. Thus a capital investment with a shorter payback period is more financially attractive than those with longer ones.

The advantage of payback analysis is that it's simple to calculate and easy to understand and use. The disadvantages are that it:

- Considers cumulative net cash flows only to the year they become positive; cash generated in subsequent years is not taken into account

Exhibit 9.5. Payback Analysis

Accounting period	Estimated net cash flow (in accounting period)	Cumulative net cash flow
Year 0	–$3,235,000	–$3,235,000
Year 1	$525,200	–$2,709,800
Year 2	$840,200	–$1,869,600
Year 3	$987,500	–$882,100
Year 4	$1,190,300	$308,200

- Treats the net cash flows generated across accounting periods as being of equal value; this is a simplifying assumption, since dollars in hand today are valued more than those that will be received in the future
- Presents results in years (to payback), not dollars; the monetary impact of the project is not quantified

Net Present Value Analysis

A more sophisticated, and better, way to evaluate the financial attractiveness of a capital project is net present value analysis; this technique overcomes the negatives of the payback approach.

The question addressed is: Does a project's estimated net cumulative cash flows (adjusted by a discount rate) exceed the initial investment made in it? If so, by how much?

The structure of net present value analysis is shown in Exhibit 9.6. All information is the same as used in payback analysis. The difference is that annual net cumulative cash flows generated in each accounting period during the project's life are discounted to their present value (at time zero) by applying a discount rate. A discount rate is an organization's estimated cost of capital; determining it is a complex process beyond the scope of this book.

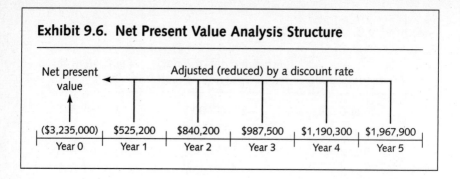

Exhibit 9.6. Net Present Value Analysis Structure

Net present value

Adjusted (reduced) by a discount rate

($3,235,000)	$525,200	$840,200	$987,500	$1,190,300	$1,967,900
Year 0	Year 1	Year 2	Year 3	Year 4	Year 5

The information needed to conduct a net present value analysis (based on Exhibit 9.4) is depicted in columns one (project life) and two (net cash flow for the accounting period) of Exhibit 9.7. The present value of future sums of money (column three) is calculated as:

$$PV = \frac{FV}{(1 + r)^t}$$

Where:

- *PV* is present value of the dollars at time zero
- *FV* is the dollar value of an estimated net cash flow in a future accounting period
- *r* is the discount rate expressed as a proportion; thus 16 percent becomes .16 (note: this figure is illustrative only and not intended to be a recommended discount rate)
- *t* is the number of years from time zero to the accounting period in which future dollars are generated

Thus the present value of the estimated net cash flow generated in year three is calculated as:

$$\frac{\$987,500}{(1.16)^3} = \$632,649$$

Essentials of Health Care Organization Finance

Net present value is calculated as the sum of present value net cash flow estimates by year over a project's life span:

$$NPV = PV_0 + PV_1 + PV_2 + PV_3 + PV_4 + PV_5$$

This is the total of column three in Exhibit 9.7 ($69,148).

Exhibit 9.7. Net Present Value Calculation

Discount rate = 16%

Column 1 Accounting period	Column 2 Net cash flow	Column 3 Present value
Year 0	($3,235,000)	($3,235,000)
Year 1	$525,200	$452,759
Year 2	$840,200	$624,405
Year 3	$987,500	$632,649
Year 4	$1,190,300	$657,392
Year 5	$1,967,900	$936,943
Net present value =		$69,148

On the basis of pure financial criteria, an organization should invest in all projects with a positive net present value because return exceeds the discount rate needed to cover inflation, opportunity costs, and project risks. Projects with higher net present values are more financially attractive than those with lower ones.

Net present value analysis is the recommended technique for financially evaluating significant capital projects.

Integrating Financial and Nonfinancial Criteria

If the financial worthiness of a potential capital project were the only thing that mattered, the decision-making process would be relatively simple, straightforward, and quantitative; a project would be undertaken solely on the basis of its payback period or net present value.

Financial worthiness, though necessary, is not sufficient taken alone. To be beneficial and viable, capital projects must pass muster with respect to two additional sets of criteria: vision and strategy.

Vision is the extent to which the project is aligned with the board-formulated vision, thereby making a contribution to meeting the needs and expectations, and furthering the interests of, the organization's stakeholders and community. Vision fit is essential; projects without a high level of fit are orphans and unsustainable. For example, an in-vitro fertilization program might be a financial "barn burner" but a poor fit with the vision of a Catholic hospital.

Strategic is the extent to which the project enhances the organization's overall sustainable advantage with respect to its competitors in the market. Such advantage might be either offensive (for example, increasing market share) or defensive (blocking attempts of competitors to increase their market share). The strategic advantage of a project may not be captured in the factors employed to undertake a purely financial analysis of a proposed capital project.

Financial worthiness can be assessed quantitatively, whereas the degree of vision fit and competitive advantage are qualitative. This presents a challenge: combining incompatible (even conflicting) methodologies and criteria to make capital investment decisions. Obviously, the most attractive projects will have a high level of vision fit, strategic advantage, and financial worthiness.

IN THE BOARDROOM

➤ Does your organization employ a narrow or broad definition of capital projects? Is it focused just on fixed assets (such as facilities and equipment) or on investments in all projects designed to produce benefits over the long run? We strongly recommend the latter.

➤ Regarding the organization's strategic and financial plans, does your board designate funds to be used exclusively for capital investments? This is an essential practice of rational and focused capital decision making and allocation.

➤ To what extent do popularity, historical, political, championship, and mimic factors influence your organization's capital investment decisions? If they are used (alone or in combination) as the primary approach, your board should have a discussion with management regarding the benefits of designing and installing a more rational and sophisticated process, the key elements of which are:

Processing and considering all but emergency projects at the same time in a batch, appropriately coordinated with the organization's strategic and financial planning and budgeting cycles

Grouping proposed projects into categories by specific criteria (we suggest their type plus the amount of resources requested)

Developing explicit, but differing, assessment and approval processes depending on category

For the most important and significant categories of projects, subjecting them to a standardized and thorough financial assessment employing either payback or net present value analysis combined with an evaluation of their vision fit and the extent to which they enhance the organization's competitive advantage

➤ Your board must develop and employ specific criteria to identify which capital investment decisions it will review and authorize, and have a well-thought-out process for doing so.

➤ It is critical that your board periodically assess:

Individual capital investment decisions to determine if stated objectives (for instance, financial, vision fit, and strategic) are being met

The overall effectiveness and efficiency of the capital evaluation, decision-making, and allocation process

➤ There are two aspects of all capital decisions: whether a project should be undertaken (capital allocation), and where the money will come from (financing). These two decisions should be addressed separately. "Go, no go" is determined first, and if it's a go then a decision is made about how the project will be financed (for instance, the mix of debt and equity).

CHAPTER 10

Financial Integrity and Credibility

OBJECTIVES

After completing this chapter, you will have a better grasp of your board's responsibility for:

- Ensuring a high level of organizational integrity and credibility regarding recording and reporting of financial information and protection and use of financial resources
- Overseeing the external audit and internal control functions

Integrity is being honest, truthful, and transparent in one's analyses, decisions, and actions. Credibility is being trusted and perceived by others as having integrity. They are two sides of the same coin; integrity is performance, credibility is perception. One can have integrity and be perceived as not credible, or be thought credible (at least for a while) and lack integrity.

> **Enron and AHERF**
>
> The Enron and AHERF (Allegheny Health, Education, and Research Foundation) debacles, along with a host of others (El Paso Natural Gas,

(Continued)

Tyco, Global Crossings, Qwest, Adelphia Communications, PhyCor, Allina, Health South), have precipitated a crisis of confidence in the accounting, finance, and governance practices of U.S. corporations, both commercial and nonprofit. If you would like to read more about what happened and why, we recommend:

- *The Role of the Board of Directors in Enron's Collapse,* Report of the U.S. Senate Committee on Investigations (July 2002).
- "The Fall of the House of AHERF, the Allegheny Bankruptcy: A Chronicle of the Hows and Whys of the Nation's Largest Non-Profit Health Care Failure," by Lawton Burns and colleagues, *Health Affairs* (Jan.–Feb. 2000), pp. 7–41.

Customers, physicians, employees, payors, vendors, lenders, and investors won't do business for long with an organization that lacks integrity and credibility. These qualities of American business (in both nonprofit and commercial corporations) have been seriously questioned thanks to front-page news coverage of a host of organizational financial shenanigans. The "poster children" are Enron, the largest corporate bankruptcy in history; and AHERF (Allegheny Health, Education, and Research Foundation), the largest nonprofit organization (and health system) bankruptcy ever.

Financial integrity and credibility begin with the board, which must create the ethical climate and convey explicit expectations to do the right things (see "It Starts at the Top"). To fulfill its responsibility for finance and discharge its oversight role, a board must ensure that:

- Accounting systems, procedures, and practices for supplying complete, accurate, and timely information are in place and functioning effectively
- Transactions are properly authorized, executed, and recorded
- Funds are used for legitimate purposes in appropriate ways
- Financial statements present fairly, in all material respects, the organization's financial position
- The organization complies with applicable laws and regulations

It Starts at the Top

The board, by design or default and either directly or indirectly, creates ethical preconditions and context. An organization's business culture can vary along a number of important dimensions.

Organization-focused	➢	Stakeholder-focused
Aggressive	➢	Conservative
Short-term orientation	➢	Long-term orientation
Following the letter of the law	➢	Abiding by the spirit of the law
Loose internal controls	➢	Tight internal controls
Obfuscation	➢	Transparency
General and vague guidelines	➢	Specific and precise guidelines

Your board must move the organization from "left" to "right" along each of these dimensions. In addition to doing all of the specific things we address in this chapter, your board must set the tone and send a clear/consistent message regarding its ethical expectations.

To do these things, a board working with management creates an audit committee, retains an external auditor and oversees the engagement, and receives analyses and recommendations from the organization's internal audit function.

AUDIT COMMITTEE

Many health care organization boards do not have an audit committee. In the past, the functions were assumed by a finance committee or the board as a whole. We strongly recommend creation of a separate standing board audit committee, for several reasons. First, external parties (bond rating and insurance agencies, lenders, large donors, and regulators) are increasingly expecting—and even demanding—them and seeing their presence as an indicator of board-level fiscal responsibility and accountability. Second, an audit committee serves as the board's center of gravity for ensuring the integrity of financial reporting and internal control, whereas the finance committee focuses on financial planning, policy formulation, and decision making. The functions of these two committees are different and best kept separate. Third, the board serving as a committee-of-the-whole may not have the time or focus to discharge the financial oversight role. An audit committee can be a powerful tool to assist a board in ensuring a high level of financial integrity and credibility.

There are a number of ways to subdivide full board and audit committee functions. The overarching principle is that the committee does the heavy lifting, performing supportive work on behalf of, and making recommendations to, the board; the full board decides and acts. That is, committees don't govern; only a board does.

With the preceding principle in mind, a board should ensure that core functions of the audit committee include:

• Making recommendations to the board regarding audit firm selection, evaluation, retention, and authorization of fees
• Conferring with the audit firm and management to understand the scope and areas of emphasis of the annual audit
• Interacting with the auditor and management to resolve issues regarding financial reporting
• Reviewing all significant financial communications to external parties, ensuring they fairly represent the organization's financial position and are prepared in accordance with generally accepted accounting principles
• Reviewing the auditor's opinion and forwarding it to the board
• Facilitating the auditor's meeting with the full board
• Serving as a point of contact for the organization's internal audit function
• Making recommendations to the board regarding initiatives that should be undertaken by management to correct any deficiencies in financial reporting and controls

Essentials of Health Care Organization Finance

To perform these functions, the audit committee should have an annual work plan; be composed only of outside, independent directors; be chaired by a director with expertise in accounting or finance; meet frequently enough to perform its work (we recommend at least four times a year); and have adequate staff support and other resources.

THE AUDIT

The annual audit is conducted by an independent certified public accountant for the board on behalf of an organization's stakeholders. The auditor is appointed by and accountable to the board, not management. The objective of an audit is to obtain an auditor's opinion as to whether management's financial statements present fairly, in all material respects, an organization's financial position.

To formulate and render its opinion, the auditor, employing generally accepted auditing standards (GAAS), engages in a host of activities:

- Examining records
- Verifying the existence and accounting value of assets (such as property, plant, equipment, cash in bank accounts, securities and other financial instruments, accounts receivable)
- Ascertaining the nature and amount of liabilities (payments owed, loans, bonds)
- Evaluating accounting principles, practices, and controls employed by management
- Reviewing estimates made by management
- Assessing the organization's financial statements

On completing the audit, the auditor issues an opinion. There are five types:

- *Adverse opinion.* The financial statements taken as a whole do not present fairly, in conformity with GAAP, the organization's financial condition. The auditor states substantive reasons for the adverse opinion and their impact on the financial statements.

- *Disclaimer of opinion.* Here the auditors state their inability to render an opinion because they were not independent. A health care organization should never receive this type of opinion since only independent auditors are to be retained.

- *Qualified opinion.* This opinion states that, except for the effects of matters described in qualifying paragraphs, the financial statements present fairly, in all material respects, the financial condition of the organization.

- *Unqualified opinion with explanatory language.* Here, an additional paragraph is added to the clean opinion (see below) intended to inform the reader of certain facts and judgments that do not affect the auditor's opinion but are deemed important to disclose. As an example, even though the auditor was responsible for the full audit, some work was performed by another firm; or there was substantial doubt about the business entity's ability to continue as an ongoing concern.

- *Unqualified, or clean, opinion.* Exhibit 10.1 illustrates an unqualified, clean audit opinion. The language does not vary among audit firms and organizations being audited. Anything in the opinion other than these three paragraphs demands an explanation.

Regarding the opinion letter and highlighted and boldfaced portions of it:

- An organization's financial statements are the responsibility of management.

- The audit firm expresses a "reasonable assurance" regarding the organization's financial statements; it is not a guarantee of their accuracy.

- The audit focuses on whether financial statements are free of material misstatements assessed through selective testing and examination; auditors do not examine every transaction, but rather sample them.

- The opinion notes that the organization's financial statements are reported in accordance with GAAP and are a fair representation of the organization's financial position.

This last point is important. An unqualified audit opinion means the organization played and portrayed its finances "by the rules" (GAAP). It says

Essentials of Health Care Organization Finance

nothing about the organization's financial performance and condition. That is, an organization could receive a clean audit opinion and be in terrible financial shape. There is one caveat: the auditor has an obligation to convey any concerns regarding the viability of the organization as an ongoing business—that is, its potential failure in the near term.

The opinion letter appears with an organization's audited financial statements (balance sheet, revenue/expense summary, and statement of cash flows) and associated footnotes. There is no description of, or comments regarding, the auditor's methods, analyses, and concerns. These matters should be discussed by the auditor with directors at an audit committee and full board meeting. Some areas that your board should explore, and questions that you might want to ask, are in Exhibit 10.2.

Exhibit 10.2. Issues That Might Be Discussed with the Auditor in a Postaudit Conference

---

Regarding the process:

• Nature and scope of the audit, including any areas of special emphasis and limitations or restrictions in addition to how conduct of the audit varied from plans and the reasons why

• Evaluation of the organization's internal control systems, procedures, and practices

• Extent to which generally accepted accounting principles were appropriately and consistently employed, including the effect of alternative methods, changes in the application of GAAP across accounting periods, and significant reporting and judgment issues made in connection with the preparation of financial statements

• Degree of cooperation received by the auditors from management in conducting the audit

• Disagreements (if any) of auditors and management and how they were resolved

• Nature of significant material errors and potential illegal acts uncovered during the audit

• Extent to which the audit firm provides consulting services to the organization, the type and nature of such engagements, and whether they might compromise the auditor's independence

• What the board should be doing (differently or better) to create the climate and conditions that would enhance the organization's financial integrity and credibility

The "big ones":

• Extent to which financial statements fully and fairly reflect the organization's financial position; what should be done to improve financial reporting and communication

Essentials of Health Care Organization Finance

Exhibit 10.2. Issues That Might Be Discussed with the Auditor in a Postaudit Conference, Cont'd.

- Nature and magnitude of financial statement variances between accounting periods in addition to the cause and their implications for the organization's financial condition
- Nature of significant adjustments made to the financial statements and footnotes as a result of the audit process

Important specifics:

- Use of complex or unusual financial transactions and instruments (such as all types of off-balance-sheet financing)
- Nature and amount of capital leases entered into by the organization, and trends over the past three years
- Areas of significant financial risk or exposure and how well they are being managed
- Reasonableness of assumptions, estimates, and judgments made by management to produce financial statements (such as contractual allowances and bad debt)
- Nature and amount of unusual prior-period adjustments and accounting accruals
- Nature of significant contingent liabilities and whether reserves have been established
- Extent to which the organization is in conformance with bond covenants
- Nature and amount of significant related-party transactions among subsidiary business units
- Type and amount of significant assets written off during the accounting period
- Nature of payments to members of the medical staff for such things as administrative salaries, relocation expenses, and rent or lease subsidies
- Nature of any nonsalary payments made to executives
- Potential problems associated with expropriation of, or the use of, restricted funds
- Effect of any mergers or acquisitions, restructurings, and dispositions of assets on the organization's financial statements and condition
- Pending legal actions and litigation that could materially affect the organization's financial condition and the reserves established

INTERNAL CONTROLS

Virtually all large commercial corporations have a formally organized internal audit function. This practice is less well established in health care organizations generally, although most medium-to-large health systems and hospitals have them. In the past, some organizations contracted with their external auditor to perform internal audit functions; we do not recommend this practice because it creates a potential conflict.

An internal audit function:

- Promotes fiscal accountability
- Monitors and assesses an organization's internal control systems, procedures, and practices
- Evaluates financial risks and exposure
- Analyzes operational efficiency
- Investigates allegations of impropriety, fraud, and abuse
- Evaluates the safety of, and appropriate access to, information systems
- Ensures compliance with laws, regulations, and the organization's own policies

There are a number of ways this function can be designed, organized, and managed. We recommend that the internal audit function have a board-approved mandate or charter defining its responsibilities and ensuring its autonomy, appropriate staffing and resources, and a direct communication channel to the board (typically through the audit committee).

EMERGING EXPECTATIONS AND STANDARDS

The post-Enron backlash against ineffective, negligent, or fraudulent governance has resulted in legislation and regulation designed to hold commercial corporation boards to much higher standards of accountability, performance, and functional transparency—particularly in the area of financial oversight. The Public Company Accounting Reform and Investor Protection (Sarbanes-Oxley) Act of 2002, and associated rules of the New

Essentials of Health Care Organization Finance

York Stock Exchange, impose requirements on public company boards with the purpose of protecting investors. You've likely read about one of the most widely reported provisions of this act, the one requiring CEOs and CFOs to personally attest to the accuracy of their organization's financial statements.

The Sarbanes-Oxley Act and NYSE rules don't apply to nonprofit organizations. However, they are being increasingly employed by bond rating and insurance agencies, lenders, regulators, accreditors, foundations, major donors, the press, and the public to assess the extent to which the boards of large nonprofits (particularly health systems and hospitals) are effectively discharging their financial responsibilities.

An executive summary of key Sarbanes-Oxley Act provisions and associated NYSE rules dealing with governance-related finance and accounting issues and board audit committees is presented in Appendix B.

Given changes in governance standards and expectations, many boards have developed a "code of conduct." Boards are increasingly recognizing that an organization's reputation is one critical determinant of its value. Explicitly stated and board endorsed ethical standards and precise guidelines regarding acceptable or unacceptable practices can be helpful in creating a climate of integrity and credibility. Of course, such a code doesn't guarantee ethical behavior; however, it is fundamental for establishing a necessary "tone at the top." To be useful, a code must:

- Be very specific, rather than a vague recitation of the importance of good corporate citizenship
- Take account of the organization's vision and circumstances
- Be a distinctive product of the board's and management's careful debate and deliberation, rather than taken off the shelf or borrowed from others
- Explicitly and precisely convey the organization's most important ethical "shoulds" and "should-nots"
- Lay out methods that can be employed to report suspected or alleged infractions

The code should be widely distributed to executives, employees, medical staff, payors, and vendors. Compliance systems must be designed and put in place, and training must occur. Illustrative code of conduct provisions are in Appendix C.

IN THE BOARDROOM

➤ Who is your organization's auditor? Some suggest that auditors should be changed about every five to seven years in order to ensure their independence. We do not recommend this as a hard-and-fast rule, but your board should have a policy regarding periodic change of audit firms. Your board must balance a firm's experience and familiarity with the organization and the decreasing objectivity that comes with long tenure. However, we suggest that the supervising audit partner be rotated periodically.

➤ If you have not done so, review the last several years of audit opinions and associated management letters.

➤ Has your organization ever received an audit opinion other than unqualified? When? What were the reasons?

➤ Does the audit firm provide consulting services to the organization? What type of work is done, and what were the fees billed over the last three years? It is not uncommon for audit firms to provide services such as tax advice and Medicare cost report review. However, we recommend that (without exception) all audit firm consulting work be approved, before the fact, by the audit committee.

➤ Does your board have a separate, standing audit committee? Does it have a charter? Is it composed totally of outside directors? Does the committee's chair have expertise in accounting or finance? If your board does not have a separate audit committee, are the functions described here performed by another board committee?

➤ Are results of the annual audit carefully reviewed by your board at a regular or special meeting where directors have adequate time to be briefed and ask questions? Is a portion of this meeting held in executive session, without management present?

➤ Does your organization have an internal audit function? If so:

What were the nature and scope of its activities during the past several years?

How is it staffed, and does it have adequate resources?

Are its objectives and work plan approved by the audit committee?

Does it communicate directly with the audit committee or board?

➤ Review the Sarbanes-Oxley and NYSE rules summarized in Appendix B. How do your organization and board stack up?

➤ Does your organization have a formal code of conduct?

CHAPTER 11

The Finale

OBJECTIVES

This chapter concludes our journey. Here we:

- Present some overarching admonitions regarding the things your board must do to fulfill its responsibility for ensuring the organization's financial health

- Present a checklist you can use to do a quick assessment of your board's financial fitness and savvy

- Recommend some resources for learning more about health care organization governance, accounting, and finance

ADMONITIONS

Here are some parting admonitions. They are the big blips that should be on your board's financial radar screen.

 • To make a difference (on behalf of stakeholders) and add value (to the organization), your board must have a coherent, precise, and shared notion of its obligation and the type of work it should be doing. Your board's overarching obligation is ensuring the organization's resources and capacities are deployed in ways that maximize community and stakeholder benefit. To fulfill this obligation, your board must formulate policy, make decisions, and oversee ends (vision, goals, and strategies), executive performance and compensation, the quality of care, and finances. Heed the wisdom of Martin Luther King, Jr.: "Keep your eyes on the prize." Do everything you can to ensure that directors define the practice of governance in the same way. This, more than anything else, focuses your board's attention and effort on those things that matter most.

- Recognize that being accountable for financial performance and condition is one of your board's most important responsibilities. Only a financially healthy organization can be an effective vehicle for serving its community and stakeholders. Strategic, operational, and clinical initiatives are fueled by money. A health care organization is among the community's most critical social institutions, but it is also a business that must be economically viable. Your board, as a steward of the community's investment, must ensure this.

- To be a faithful financial steward, your board must:

   Set financial direction, objectives, and policy

   Ensure that effective financial planning and capital allocation systems are in place and functioning effectively

   Question and test the soundness of financial plans and capital investment proposals

   Ensure that strategic, operational, and financial plans and decisions maintain and enhance the organization's creditworthiness

   Monitor and assess the organization's financial performance

   Ensure that financial statements fairly reflect the organization's condition and that funds are being deployed for appropriate purposes in legitimate ways

Keep in mind that your board's job is to make sure the organization is financially well managed, *not* to financially manage it. For example, if your board becomes aware of a financial problem, your responsibility is to understand it and frame expectations; management's responsibility is to solve it.

- The effectiveness and efficiency of your board depends, in no small measure, on the information it receives—the right kind in the right form and format at the right time. The type of financial information your board needs to govern is very different from what executives require to manage. Expect management to provide governance-focused and friendly information consciously and specifically crafted to assist your board in fulfilling its responsibilities:

Production of custom-designed, nontraditional financial statements that are easy for directors to read and interpret

A streamlined and consistent way of presenting financial information and talking through the numbers at board and finance committee meetings

Standardized, graphical dashboards (including indicators and benchmarks) employed by your board to continuously monitor and assess the organization's financial performance and condition

- It's virtually impossible for your board to fulfill its responsibilities, without having appropriately configured and functioning finance and audit committees. Ensure that these committees:

Do governance-related staff work that focuses and leverages the board's time and effort when it meets; only the full board, not its committees, governs, formulates policies, and makes decisions

Have charters specifying committee objectives, functions, deliverables, membership, and the nature of staff support

Are chaired by, and have members with, knowledge and experience in accounting and finance

The finance committee should vet the financial aspects of every significant management proposal before it is placed on the board's agenda. The audit committee should be composed of outside (independent) directors and should hold some of its meetings without management present.

- Your board should consider developing a financial calendar (see Exhibit 11.1 for an illustration). This is a great planning tool and schedules

Exhibit 11.1. Illustrative Board Financial Calendar

	Audit committee (meets four times per year)	Finance committee (meets every other month)	Full board (meets monthly)
January		• Overview and discussion of current financial performance; transmittal of issues to the full board as warranted • Service line reports • Year-end review of financial statements (unaudited) • Review of investment performance • Investment policy review	• Investment policy review and approval • Year-end financial review (unaudited)
February			• CEO/CFO presentation; brief review of financial performance
March	• Internal auditor's report • Internal control report • Review and approve internal control workplan	• Overview and discussion of current financial performance; transmittal of issues to the full board as warranted • Service line reports • Accounts receivable review (revenue cycle, credit policy, charity policy) • Community benefits assessment	• CEO/CFO presentation; brief review of financial performance • Review and approval of credit and charity policies • Review of community benefits

Month		
April	• External auditor's presentation; discussion, questions, and comments • Executive session with auditor • Evaluation of audit and auditor	• External auditor's presentation; discussion, questions, and commentary • Executive session with auditor • Appoint or reappoint external auditor; approve fees
May	• Overview and discussion of current financial performance; transmittal of issues to the full board as warranted • Long-range financial plan update and review • Budget goals and targets for next year	• CEO/CFO presentation; brief review of financial performance and condition • Review and approve budget targets for forthcoming year
June	• Internal auditor's report • Review and comment: internal audit work plan • Internal control report • Review of external reporting (bond trustees, rating agencies, cost reports)	• Review and approve internal auditor work plan
July	• Overview and discussion of current financial performance; transmittal of issues to the full board as warranted • Service line reports • Comprehensive financial review (six months, year to date) • Review of budget assumptions	• Comprehensive financial review (six months, year to date)

(Continued)

Exhibit 11.1. Illustrative Board Financial Calendar, Cont'd.

	Audit committee (meets four times per year)	Finance committee (meets every other month)	Full board (meets monthly)
August			
September		• Overview and discussion of current financial performance; transmittal of issues to the full board as warranted • Service line reports • Third-party payor contracting update • Medicare and Medicaid legislation and regulation update	• CEO/CFO presentation; brief review of financial performance
October			
November	• Audit planning • Internal auditor's report • Internal control report • Review of external reporting (bond trustees and rating agencies)	• Overview and discussion of current financial performance; transmittal of issues to the full board as warranted • Review and accept budget • Long-range financial plan update	• Review and accept budget • Long-range financial plan update and review
December			• CEO/CFO presentation; brief review of financial performance

key, routine, nonemergency tasks that must be undertaken by the finance committee, audit committee, and full board throughout the year.

- Your board should expect management to engage in state-of-the-art financial planning and budgeting. Once a luxury, this is needed to deal with an increasingly competitive industry and local markets in addition to far larger and much more complex organizations.

- Health care organization access to debt financing at reasonable rates is more problematic than in the past because of increasingly stringent expectations on the part of lenders. Your board must constantly keep its eye on the organization's creditworthiness. We believe a key governance practice for doing so is board-set financial objectives and benchmarks keyed to specific ratio values that must be achieved to secure a targeted bond rating.

- How much capital is available to invest in the organization and the way in which it is allocated across projects define and determine its future. Your board must ensure that management has a coherent and effective process for doing so, based on corporate finance principles.

- In times past, board oversight and approval of the audit was pretty much a "pass" and passive. In this arena, board responsibility has changed dramatically thanks to a host of organizational debacles, audit firm improprieties, and increased expectations and standards being imposed by bond rating agencies, institutional lenders, and major donors. Your board is ultimately accountable for ensuring that the organization's financial statements fairly reflect its financial status. The external auditor is chosen by, and reports to, your board (not management). Your board (with heavy lifting done by the audit committee) must take this responsibility seriously and put in place policies and processes (including a well-designed and autonomous internal audit function and an explicit, enforceable code of ethics) to safeguard the organization's financial integrity and credibility.

- Recognize that the nature and quality of relationships among your board, CEO, and CFO are critical ingredients for effective performance of governance financial work (policy formulation, decision making, and oversight), and ultimately the organization's long-run financial health. To work well on behalf of stakeholders, the community, and the organization, this relationship must be characterized by:

A clear and mutually empowering subdivision of accountabilities and responsibilities

A free flow of information

Honest and straightforward discussion and deliberation

Trust (based on the experience of seeing expectations and commitments fulfilled)

Empathy and respect

Your board should expect management to be proactive in addressing its potential concerns, questions, and needs for information. We are not suggesting the CEO and CFO become mind readers; however, they should identify issues that might concern the board, frame them, and be prepared to recommend solutions—before being asked to do so. Additionally, your board, the CEO, and the CFO should work with one another employing the doctrine of no surprises: striving for reasonable predictability, and when unanticipated problems arise, getting them on the table for discussion quickly.

- We recommend that the board, with the assistance of a qualified consultant, undertake a thorough assessment of the organization's financial performance and condition every several years (recall that the annual audit does not do this). An outside set of eyes can be a board's best check that it's aware of any potential problems and fulfilling its responsibility for ensuring the organization's financial health. Dennis M. Stillman Associates works with boards on such engagements and can be reached at (206) 459-1846 or stillmanassoc@w-link.net.

- By reading this book, you have acquired basic financial literacy. With knowledge comes the confidence that's essential for probing, asking tough questions, monitoring the organization's performance and condition, and understanding management's financial plans. But governance is a team sport. Your director colleagues must also be up to speed for the board to collectively fulfill its foundational responsibility of ensuring the organization's financial health.

CHECKLIST

Governance financial fitness and savvy do not come easily; to achieve them, your board must have the right stuff in place and do the right things well. To summarize many of the most important ideas forwarded in the book, here's a checklist. How does your board stack up?

✓ My board has identified the organization's key stakeholders and mapped their most important interests, needs, and expectations.
☐ yes ☐ somewhat ☐ no

✓ Directors have a shared and coherent understanding of the nature of our board's governance work—its obligations, responsibilities, and roles.
☐ yes ☐ somewhat ☐ no

✓ All directors understand the basics of health care organization accounting and finance.
☐ yes ☐ somewhat ☐ no

✓ At least one director has highly developed financial expertise and experience.
☐ yes ☐ somewhat ☐ no

✓ At least annually, my board is updated on significant trends in, and major threats and opportunities posed by, the health care industry, our local market(s), and competitors.
☐ yes ☐ somewhat ☐ no

✓ Annually, my board formulates precise and explicit financial objectives for the organization.
☐ yes ☐ somewhat ☐ no

✓ Our board has a standing finance committee.
☐ yes ☐ somewhat ☐ no

✓ The finance committee:
☐ yes ☐ somewhat ☐ no

   Is chaired by a director with knowledge and experience in finance

Reviews, evaluates, and makes recommendations regarding all major finance-
related policies and decisions coming
before our board for discussion and vote

Annually prepares an analysis of the
organization's financial performance
and condition for full board review,
discussion, and action

✓ Financial statements presented to my board
are governance-friendly; they are easy to
read and interpret.

☐ yes	☐ somewhat	☐ no

✓ At least twice each year, on the basis of
preparatory work undertaken by the finance
committee, my board reviews and assesses
the revenue and expense summary, balance
sheet, and statement of cash flows.

☐ yes	☐ somewhat	☐ no

✓ (For health care systems) my board is given
consolidated financial statements in addition to those for all subsidiary organizations.

☐ yes	☐ somewhat	☐ no

✓ My board uses a financial dashboard system
to assist in discharging its oversight role;
the dashboard is composed of liquidity,
profitability, capital structure, activity, and
operating ratios and statistics either selected
individually or tied to a board-specified
bond rating target.

☐ yes	☐ somewhat	☐ no

✓ At least quarterly, from analyses prepared
by the finance committee, my board reviews
the extent to which the organization is
meeting board-specified financial objectives,
and its financial performance and condition
as reflected by dashboard indicators.

☐ yes	☐ somewhat	☐ no

✓ My board has formulated a fine-grained, explicit, and empowering vision that specifies what the organization should become in the future to maximize stakeholder benefit; this vision is reviewed (and modified, if needed) annually.

☐ yes ☐ somewhat ☐ no

✓ Annually, my board reviews and approves core organizational strategies developed by management, ensuring they are aligned with the board-formulated vision.

☐ yes ☐ somewhat ☐ no

✓ Annually, management prepares a rolling five-to-eight-year financial plan that contains: a specification of assumptions and estimates; pro forma financial statements and ratio, horizontal, and vertical analyses; and an assessment of vulnerabilities and risks.

☐ yes ☐ somewhat ☐ no

✓ Annually, grounded in preparatory work by the finance committee, my board reviews, discusses, and approves management's financial plan, ensuring it is aligned with the vision and strategic plan.

☐ yes ☐ somewhat ☐ no

✓ Annually, management prepares a budget (with statistical, revenue, expense, capital, and cash components) for the organization (and in a health system for each subsidiary).

☐ yes ☐ somewhat ☐ no

✓ On the basis of preparatory work by the finance committee, summaries and analyses of significant budget variances are reviewed and discussed by my board.

☐ yes ☐ somewhat ☐ no

✓ Annually, with input from management and our investment banker, my board reviews

☐ yes ☐ somewhat ☐ no

and assesses the organization's capital structure and creditworthiness.

✓ Annually, the finance committee reviews all bond covenants and ensures they are being met.

☐	☐	☐
yes	somewhat	no

✓ Using strategic and financial plans, my board designates a pool of funds (for both the current and future accounting periods) to meet the organization's long-term capital investment needs.

☐	☐	☐
yes	somewhat	no

✓ A capital project evaluation and approval process is in place that:

☐	☐	☐
yes	somewhat	no

Considers all nonemergency projects at the same time

Combines like-type projects into categories according to their risk

Subjects all proposals in a particular risk category to standardized evaluation and approval criteria

Employs payback or net present value analysis to assess project financial attractiveness

Combines financial analyses with vision fit and competitiveness assessments

✓ My board has established specific criteria to identify capital projects that require our review and approval.

☐	☐	☐
yes	somewhat	no

✓ Annually, my board assesses the extent to which previously approved major capital projects are meeting their objectives.

☐	☐	☐
yes	somewhat	no

Essentials of Health Care Organization Finance

✓ Annually, my board reviews the effectiveness
and efficiency of the organization's capital
evaluation and allocation process.

☐ yes ☐ somewhat ☐ no

✓ My board has a separate standing audit
committee, which:

☐ yes ☐ somewhat ☐ no

> Is composed totally of outside
> (nonmanagement) directors
>
> Is chaired by a director with knowledge
> and experience in accounting and finance
>
> Regularly meets without management
> present

✓ Annually, on the basis of preparatory work
undertaken by the audit committee, rep-
resentatives of the audit firm meet with
my board to:

☐ yes ☐ somewhat ☐ no

> Review the audit, audit opinion, and
> management letter
>
> Share observations and concerns and
> answer questions
>
> Discuss implications

A portion of the meeting is devoted to
executive session without management
present.

✓ The organization has an internal audit
function, which reports to my board
directly through the audit committee.

☐ yes ☐ somewhat ☐ no

✓ Management, with input and support
from my board, has formulated a code of
ethics.

☐ yes ☐ somewhat ☐ no

RESOURCES

If you want to increase your governance and financial knowledge and competencies beyond what you've learned by reading this book, here are some recommendations.

Dennis D. Pointer & Associates conducts one-day "financial boot camps" for groups of health care organization directors. They can be sponsored by individual health care organizations, state or local hospital associations, or professional associations. For information, call (206) 632–6066 or e-mail dennis.pointer@comcast.net.

To learn more about health care organization boards and governance, we recommend:

Board Work, by Dennis Pointer and James Orlikoff (Jossey-Bass, 1999), 291 pages. Winner of the James A. Hamilton Book of the Year award from the American College of Healthcare Executives.

Getting to Great: Principles of Health Care Organization Governance, by Dennis Pointer and James Orlikoff (Jossey-Bass, 2002), 202 pages.

Boards That Make a Difference, by John Carver (Jossey-Bass, 1997), 241 pages.

These books can be ordered by calling Jossey-Bass at (888) 378–2537.

Directors must understand the context in which the organization they govern operates. Here is a good overview: *The Health Care Industry: A Primer for Board Members,* by Dennis Pointer and Stephen Williams (Jossey-Bass, 2003), 135 pages.

Ask your CEO to enter magazine and newsletter subscriptions for you and your fellow directors. We recommend:

Modern Healthcare (888/446–1422; www.modernhealthcare.com). This is the premier weekly health care industry news source. The magazine is targeted at executives, but it's an excellent resource for directors.

Trustee Magazine (800/621–6920; www.trusteemag.com). Published by the American Hospital Association for health care organization directors.

American Governance Leader (866/342–5245; www.americangovernance
.com). This is a monthly newsletter for health care organization directors that focuses on both the process of governing and the substantive
issues with which boards must deal.

For a more comprehensive and in-depth treatment of managerial accounting and finance, we recommend:

Finance in Brief: Six Key Concepts for Healthcare Leaders, by Kenneth
Kaufman (Health Administration Press, 2000), 105 pages. This book is
focused on the capital management cycle and targeted at nonspecialists.
*Healthcare Finance: An Introduction to Accounting and Financial
Management,* by Louis Gapenski (Health Administration Press, 1999),
555 pages. This is one of the best accounting or finance texts for graduate students in health administration; it has been adopted by many
programs (including ours at the University of Washington). If you want
more depth, this should be your next step.

Here are Websites for some organizations mentioned in the text:

> www.aicpa.org (American Institute of Certified Public Accountants)
>
> www.hfma.org (Healthcare Financial Management Association)
>
> www.moodys.com (Moody's Investors Service)
>
> www.standardandpoors.com (Standard & Poor's)
>
> www.fitchratings.com (FitchRating Service)

There are a number of governance development and resource Websites;
among the best:

> www.americangovernance.com (American Governance and
> Leadership Group)
>
> www.boardsource.org (formerly the National Center for Nonprofit
> Boards)
>
> www.naconline.org (National Association of Corporate Directors)

www.angonline.org (Alliance for Nonprofit Governance)

www.nonprofitresourcectr.org (Nonprofit Resource Center)

www.calpers-governance.org (California Public Employees' Retirement System governance resource site; CalPers is the nation's largest pension fund and has been a leader in promoting principle-based governance)

www.corpgov.hbs.edu (Corporate Governance Initiative of Harvard University's School of Business)

http://iicg.som.yale.edu (International Institute for Corporate Governance of Yale University's School of Management)

E. Polley Francis Hospital, Traditionally Configured Financial Statements

Exhibit A.1.
E. Polley Francis Hospital
Revenue and Expense Summary
for the Year Ending December 31, 2006,
by Natural Class of Expense
(000)

Revenue

Unrestricted revenues and other operating revenue:

Net patient services revenue	$323,100
Other revenue	17,600
Total revenue	$340,700

Expenses

Salaries and wages	$118,500
Benefits and taxes	39,500
Supplies, drugs, prostheses, and other	138,500
Depreciation	20,667
Interest expense	3,400
Allowance for bad debts	7,300
Total expenses	$327,867
Net income from operations	$12,833
Nonoperating revenues	$11,415
Nonoperating expenses	2,500
Net nonoperating income	$8,915
Excess of revenue over expenses	$21,748

Note: This revenue and expense summary is organized by natural class of expense.

Exhibit A.2.
E. Polley Francis Hospital
Revenue and Expense Summary
for the Year Ending December 31, 2006,
by Service
(000)

Revenue

Unrestricted revenues and other operating revenue:

Net patient services revenue	$323,100
Other revenue	17,600
Total revenue	$340,700

Expenses

Patient care	$131,200
Ancillary	65,600
Support	49,200
Administrative	57,767
Depreciation and interest	24,100
Total expenses	$327,867
Net income from operations	$12,833
Nonoperating revenues	$11,415
Nonoperating expenses	2,500
Net nonoperating income	$8,915
Excess of revenue over expenses	$21,748

Note: This revenue and expense summary is organized by service.

Exhibit A.3.
E. Polley Francis Hospital
Balance Sheet,
December 31, 2006
(000)

Assets		Liabilities and net assets	
Current assets		**Current liabilities**	
Cash	$8,000	Accrued payroll	$12,000
Marketable securities	11,000	Accrued benefits and taxes	5,400
Short-term investments	19,200	Accounts payable	29,900
Patient accounts receivable, net		Current portion of long-term debt	4,300
of allowance for doubtful accounts	67,900	Payable to agencies	17,180
Inventories	6,600	Total current liabilities	$68,780
Other current assets	1,100		
Total current assets	$113,800	Long-term debt, net of current portion	48,800
		Total liabilities	$117,580
Assets whose use is limited:			
Board-designated for building	$38,595	**Net assets:**	
Trustee-held funds, bond reserve	6,000	Unrestricted	$215,735
Long-term investments	50,000	Temporarily restricted	9,900
Capital assets, at cost, net of		Permanently restricted	25,000
accumulated depreciation	159,820	Total net assets	$250,635
Total noncurrent assets	$254,415		
Total assets	$368,215	**Total liabilities and net assets**	$368,215

Exhibit A.4.
E. Polley Francis Hospital
Statement of Cash Flows
for the Year Ending December 31, 2006
(000)

Cash flows from operating activities:	
Revenue in excess of expenses	$21,748
Adjustments to reconcile change in net assets	
to net cash provided by operating activities:	
Depreciation and amortization	20,667
Change in patient accounts receivable	(2,500)
Change in inventories and other current assets	300
Change in accrued payroll, benefits, and taxes	1,400
Change in accounts payable	4,800
Change in payables to agencies	(11,620)
Net cash provided by operating activities	$34,795
Cash flows from investing activities:	
Purchase of investments	$(5,395)
Capital expenditures	(25,620)
Net cash provided by investing activities	$(31,015)
Cash flows from financing activities:	
Payments on long-term debt	$(3,500)
Payments on capital lease obligations	(200)
Contribution from parent organization	1,720
Net cash provided by financing activities	$(1,980)
Net increase (decrease) in cash and cash equivalents	$1,800
Cash and cash equivalents, beginning of year	6,200
Cash and cash equivalents, end of year	$8,000

Executive Summary of Sarbanes-Oxley Act Provisions and NYSE Governance Rules

The backlash from Enron and AHERF against ineffective, negligent, and fraudulent governance has resulted in recent legislation and regulations designed to hold commercial corporation boards to much higher standards of accountability, performance, and functional transparency. Specifically, the Public Company Accounting Reform and Investor Protection Act of 2002 (called the Sarbanes-Oxley Act) and the New York Stock Exchange's corporate governance rules impose new, and far more stringent, requirements on public company boards.

Although the law and derivative NYSE rules are not applicable to nonprofit organizations, it is likely they will form the foundation of expectations and establish a framework for future legislation and case law affecting health care boards. Additionally, such standards will be increasingly embraced by accrediting bodies, bond rating agencies and insurers, major donors, and the public.

A summary of key provisions (adapted from the Act and rules) follows.

- *Companies must have a majority of independent directors.* To be deemed "independent," the board must determine that a director has no material relationship with the company (either directly or as a partner, shareholder, or officer of an organization that has a relationship with the company).
- *Nonmanagement directors of each company must meet at regularly scheduled executive sessions without management.*
- *Companies must establish a compensation committee composed entirely of independent directors.* The committee must have a written charter that addresses:

> The committee's purpose, which, at a minimum, must be to (1) discharge the board's responsibilities relating to compensation of the company's executives and (2) produce an annual report on executive compensation for inclusion in the company's proxy statement
>
> The committee's duties and responsibilities, which, at a minimum, must be to (1) review and approve corporate goals and objectives relevant to CEO compensation, evaluate the CEO's performance in light of those goals and objectives, and set the CEO's compensation level according to this evaluation; and (2) make recommendations to the board with respect to incentive-compensation plans and equity-based plans
>
> An annual performance evaluation of the compensation committee
>
> Committee member qualifications
>
> Committee member appointment and removal
>
> Committee structure and operations (including authority to delegate to subcommittees)
>
> Reporting to the board

Under this rule, the charter must grant the committee sole authority to retain and terminate any consulting firm engaged to assist in evaluating director, CEO, or senior executive compensation, including the sole authority to approve the firm's fees and other retention terms. A board may delegate responsibilities of this committee to another committee of its choosing; this committee, however, must be composed entirely of independent directors and must have a published committee charter.

- The audit committee must be composed entirely of independent directors who must be financially literate or who become so within a reasonable period of time after appointment. The NYSE rule notes that the functions of the audit committee may not be delegated to another committee.

- At least one member of the audit committee must have a high level of accounting or related financial management expertise. In defining the term *financial expert,* the board must consider whether a person has, through education and experience:

> An understanding of GAAP and financial statements
>
> Experience in preparing or auditing financial statements of generally comparable issuers, and applying such principles in connection with the accounting for estimates, accruals, and reserves
>
> Experience with internal accounting controls
>
> An understanding of audit committee functions

- The audit committee must adopt a written charter that, at a minimum, addresses:

> Board oversight of (1) the integrity of the company's financial statements, (2) the company's compliance with legal and regulatory requirements, (3) the independent auditor's qualifications and independence, and (4) the performance of the company's internal audit function and independent auditors
>
> Preparation of the report that SEC rules require to be included in the company's annual proxy statement
>
> The duties and responsibilities of the audit committee

This rule requires the audit committee have the sole authority to approve all audit engagement fees and terms, as well as all significant nonaudit engagements with the independent auditors. These responsibilities may not be delegated to management; the committee, however, may consult with management regarding these matters.

- *The audit committee must, at least annually, obtain and review a report by the independent auditor.* The report should describe:

> The auditor's internal quality-control procedures

> Any material issues raised by the most recent internal quality control review, or peer review, of the auditor, or by any inquiry or investigation by governmental or professional authorities, within the preceding five years, and any steps taken to deal with any such issues

> All relationships between the independent auditor and the company

This assessment should include an evaluation of the lead partner on the audit. In making its evaluation, the audit committee should take into account the opinions of management and the company's internal auditors (or other personnel responsible for the internal audit function). In addition to ensuring regular rotation of the lead audit partner as required by law, the audit committee must consider whether there should be regular rotation of the audit firm itself. The audit committee should present its conclusions to the full board.

- The audit committee must review with the independent auditor any audit problems or difficulties and management's response. This rule requires the audit committee to regularly review with the independent auditor any difficulties the auditor encountered in the course of the audit work, including any restrictions on the scope of the independent auditor's activities or access to requested information, and any significant disagreements with management. Among the items the audit committee should review with the auditor are:

> Any accounting adjustments that were noted or proposed by the auditor but were "passed" (as immaterial or otherwise)

Any communications between the audit team and the audit firm's national office respecting auditing or accounting issues presented by the engagement

Any "management" or "internal control" letters issued, or proposed to be issued, by the audit firm to the company

The responsibilities, budget, and staffing of the company's internal audit function

- *The audit committee must, as needed, obtain advice and assistance from outside legal, accounting, or other advisors.*
- *The audit committee must discuss policies with respect to risk assessment and risk management.* The audit committee must address guidelines and policies to govern the process by which risk assessment and risk management is handled. The audit committee should discuss the company's major financial risk exposures and steps management has taken to monitor and control such exposures.
- *The audit committee must meet separately, periodically, with management, internal auditors (or other personnel responsible for the internal audit function), and independent auditors.*
- *The audit committee must report regularly to the board of directors.* The audit committee must review with the full board any issues that arise with respect to (1) the quality or integrity of the company's financial statements, (2) the company's compliance with legal or regulatory requirements, (3) the performance and independence of the company's independent auditors, and (4) the performance of the internal audit function.
- *The audit committee must conduct an annual performance evaluation of the company.* The audit committee must review (1) major issues regarding accounting principles and financial statement presentations, including any significant changes in the company's selection or application of accounting principles, and major issues as to the adequacy of the company's internal controls and any special audit steps adopted in light of material control deficiencies; (2) analyses prepared by management or the independent auditor setting forth significant financial reporting issues and judgments made

in connection with the preparation of the financial statements, including analyses of the effects of alternative GAAP methods on the financial statements; (3) the effect of regulatory and accounting initiatives, as well as off-balance-sheet structures, on the financial statements of the company; and (4) earnings press releases (paying particular attention to any use of "pro forma," or "adjusted" non-GAAP information), as well as financial information and earnings guidance provided to analysts and rating agencies.

- *Each listed company must have an internal audit function.* This rule does not require a company to establish a separate internal audit department or dedicate employees to the task on a full-time basis. All a company needs is to have in place an appropriate control process for reviewing and approving its internal transactions and accounting. This function may be outsourced to a firm other than its independent auditor.

- *Companies must adopt and disclose a code of business conduct and ethics for directors, officers, and employees.* Any waiver of the code for executive officers or directors may be made only by the board or a board committee and must be promptly disclosed to shareholders. Under the rule, this code should address, among others, these topics:

> Conflicts of interest. A conflict of interest occurs when an individual's private interest interferes—or even appears to interfere—with the interests of the corporation as a whole. Under the rule, each company must have a policy prohibiting conflicts of interest; this policy should also provide a way for employees, officers, and directors to communicate potential conflicts to the company.

> Corporate opportunities. Employees, officers, and directors should be prohibited from (1) taking for themselves opportunities that are discovered through the use of corporate property, information, or position; (2) using corporate property, information, or position for personal gain; and (3) competing with the company.

> Confidentiality. Confidential information entrusted to employees, officers, and directors by the company or its customers should remain so except when disclosure is authorized or legally mandated.

The rule provides that confidential information includes all non-public information that might be of use to competitors, or harmful to the company or its customers, if disclosed.

Fair dealing. No employee, officer, or director should take unfair advantage of anyone through manipulation, concealment, abuse of privileged information, misrepresentation of material facts, or any other unfair-dealing practice.

Protection and proper use of company assets. All employees, officers, and directors should protect the company's assets and ensure their efficient use.

Compliance with laws, rules, and regulations (including insider trading laws). The company should proactively promote compliance with laws, rules, and regulations, including insider trading laws, with violations of such insider trading rules being dealt with decisively.

Encouraging reporting of any illegal or unethical behavior. Employees should be encouraged to (1) talk with supervisors or managers about possible violations and (2) report violations of laws, rules, regulations, or the code of business conduct to appropriate personnel. Employees must be advised that the company will not allow retaliation for reports made in good faith. (It should be noted that under Section 806 of the Sarbanes-Oxley Act, a "whistleblower" is protected from job-related discrimination when he or she assists in the investigation of his or her employer. In addition, Section 1107 of the act imposes criminal penalties on persons who take harmful action with respect to an informant who divulges truthful information about the commission of a federal crime to a law enforcement officer.)

- Each company CEO must certify to the NYSE each year that he or she is not aware of any violation by the company of NYSE corporate governance listing standards.

E. Polley Francis Hospital, Illustrative Code-of-Conduct Provisions

- Executives are expected to make decisions that furthers EPFH's (E. Polley Francis Hospital's) long-run financial performance and health, not short-term results.

- In all of your dealings on behalf of EPFH, you are expected to decide and act in ways that abide by the letter and spirit of the law, applicable regulations, this code of conduct, and the hospital's policies; and meet the highest standards of honesty and fairness. The ultimate test is, Would you be proud of your decision or action if it were described on the front page of [name of local paper]?

- You must not accept any gifts, inducements, or benefits, the receipt of which might in any way tend to influence, or appear to influence discharging your responsibilities and duties. You should avoid all situations in which the appearance may be created that any person or organization is attempting to secure influence with, or the favor of, you or EPFH. Gifts or benefits are rarely offered by companies where the giver does not expect to receive some advantage, and you should be wary of accepting any such offers.

- If you work full-time at EPFH and wish to engage in any outside compensated employment or business activities, you are required to seek the approval of [insert office]. The approval will not be unreasonably withheld. EPFH can request the details of outside employment or compensation if they appear to pose a conflict of interest.

- It is unethical and a crime to file false claims with the Medicare and Medicaid programs or any other payors. All EPFH personnel must be extremely careful to ensure that billings to payors are prepared and submitted in strict compliance with all policies and procedures. Employees should never file or make claims for reimbursement for services that were not provided or medically unnecessary. Employees should never submit claims that contain false or misleading information. EPFH personnel have an affirmative obligation to accurately record and present information submitted to payors. EPFH will continuously conduct education programs and engage in auditing and monitoring activities related to such policies. All employees and agents with responsibility for claims development or submission are responsible for understanding and following relevant standards. If you become aware of a situation in which a false claim has been made, it should be immediately reported to [name of office].

- Antikickback laws and regulations prohibit relationships where a payment is made in exchange for referral of business. Employees must never make an offer of payment or compensation of any kind in exchange for patient referrals to EPFH. Antikickback laws and regulations provide certain "safe harbors" (exclusions and protections). It is not your responsibility to know all of these rules in detail. However, you should be cautious about any arrangements, even informal, that might be suspicious, and seek guidance from [name of office] when in doubt.

INDEX

A

Accounting basics: accounting entity, 32–33; accounting equations, 36–37; accounting period, 33; accounting principles, 32; accounting value, 36; accrual accounting, 34; conservatism, consistency, and comparability financial reporting, 35–36; expenses and depreciation, 38–40e, 39e; full disclosure and transparency, 35; importance of, 31–32; materiality, 35; monetary unit, 34; objectivity, 34; revenues, 38. *See also* Financial statements

Accounting equations: assets, 36–37, 98; average age of plant, 73; balance sheet, 53–54e; calculating days of cash on hand, 67; days revenue in accounts receivable ratio, 68; debt service coverage, 72; debt-to-equity, 71, 98; financial "ground zero," 36; financial ratio, 65; liabilities, 37; liquidity ratios, 66; net present value calculations, 122–123; operating margin, 69; owners equity, 37; payback analysis, 120; present value of future sums of money, 122; total assets turnover, 72; total margin, 69

Accounts payable, 52

Accrual accounting, 34

Accumulated depreciation, 51

Activity ratios, 72–73

Adverse opinion, 131

AHERF (Allegheny Health, Education, and Research Foundation), 127, 128

AICPA (American Institute of Certified Public Accountants), 32

American College of Healthcare Executives, 154

American Governance Leader, 155

Assets: accounting equation of, 36–37, 98; balance sheet listing current, 50; balance sheets listing noncurrent, 50–51; depreciation of, 39e–40e; PPE (property, plant, and equipment) or fixed, 51; total, 51

Audit: described, 131; as financial control, 16; five types of opinion letters following, 131–134

Audit committee, 129–131, 143

Auditors: five types of opinions issued by, 131–134; postaudit conference discussion with, 134e–135e

Average age of plant, 73

B

Bad debt (provision for uncollectables), 48

Balance sheet: accounting equation of, 53–54e; boardroom activities regarding, 57–58; described, 48–49e, 50; EPFH example of, 48–49e, 50–54e, 61e; information listed on left side of, 49e, 50–51; information listed on right side of, 49e, 51–53; summary of, 53–54e

Baylor Hospital (Texas), 25

Best effort broker relationship, 105

Blue Cross, 25

Current liabilities, 51–52
Current portions of long-term debt, 52
Current ratio, 66

D

"Dashboard" system, 76, 78
Days of cash on hand, 67
Days revenue in accounts receivable ratio,
    67–68
Debenture, 106
Debt: balance sheet listing of long-term,
    52–53; as financing source, 98; increase
    of risk due to, 99; provision for uncol-
    lectables or bad, 48
Debt service coverage, 71–72
Debt-to-equity ratio: capital structure
    quantified by, 98; described, 71; lever-
    age and, 99
Decision making: examples of board, 7;
    four options of board, 6
Dennis D. Pointer & Associates, 154
Dennis M. Stillman Associates, 148
Depreciation: accumulated, 51; calculat-
    ing asset, 40e; calculating average age
    of plant, 73; described, 39e
Disclaimer of opinion, 132
Discount rate, 118
DRGs (diagnosis-related groups):
    described, 27; Medicare flat rate of
    payment for, 46

E

Ending cash balance, 55
Enron, 127
EPFH (E. Polley Francis Hospital): aver-
    age age of plant for, 73; balance sheet
    for, 48–49e, 50–54e, 61e; capital struc-
    ture of, 98–99; current ratio of, 66;
    days in accounts receivable for, 68;
    days of cash on hand for, 67; debt
    service coverage of, 72; debt-to-equity,
    71; financial statements used by,
    43–44; horizontal and vertical finan-
    cial analyses of, 62–63e, 64e–65; net
    income or bottom line of, 48; net
    income from operations of, 48; net

nonoperating income of, 48; operating
    expenses of, 47–48; operating margin
    of, 70; operating statistics of, 74e;
    return on equity of, 70–71; revenue
    from operations of, 46, 47; revenue/
    expense summary of, 45e, 60e; state-
    ment of cash flows for, 55e, 62e; total
    assets turnover for, 73; unqualified
    audit opinion letter issued for, 133e;
    vision of, 82, 85e; working capital cal-
    culated for, 52. *See also* Financial state-
    ment analysis; Financial statements
Equity. *See* Owners equity
Executive performance responsibility, 4
Expansion capital projects, 115
Expense budget component, 94
Expenses: boardroom activities regarding,
    57; defining, 38–39; depreciation,
    39e–40e; EPFH revenue/expense sum-
    mary, 45e, 60e; financial statements on
    operating, 47–48

F

"The Fall of the House of AHERF, the
    Allegheny Bankruptcy" (Burns and
    Colleagues), 128
Feasibility consultant, 106
Fiduciary duty of loyalty of, 3
*Finance in Brief: Six Key Concepts for
    Healthcare Leaders* (Kaufman), 155
Finance committee, 16–17, 143
"Financial boot camps" (Dennis D. Pointer
    & Associates), 154
Financial calendar, 143, 144e–146e, 147
Financial integrity/credibility: audit com-
    mittee role in, 129–131; board actions
    to ensure, 128–129; boardroom activi-
    ties associated with, 138–139; emerg-
    ing expectations and standards of,
    136–138; internal controls to ensure,
    136; public debacles over, 127–128
Financial planning: assumptions and esti-
    mates used in, 91–93; benefits of,
    87–88; described, 87; example of com-
    ponents and relationships in, 91e; as
    juxtaposing financial needs with

capacity, 88–90*e*, 89*e*; long-range, 88. *See also* Budgeting

Financial responsibilities: boardroom activities associated with, 17–18; controls and audit as, 16; core board, 4, 12–13; using "dashboard" system to fulfill, 76, 78; the frog in water syndrome and, 77; key components and relationships, 13*e*; key relationships regarding, 41*e*; monitoring and assessing as, 15–16; objectives of, 13–14; organization/finance committee used to fulfill, 16–17; planning as, 15

Financial statement analysis: boardroom activities associated with, 79; financial oversight using, 76–77*e*, 78; horizontal and vertical, 62, 64*e*–65; ratio analysis, 65–76; three types of, 60. *See also* EPFH (E. Polley Francis Hospital)

Financial statements: analyzing, 59–79; balance sheet, 48–49*e*, 50–54*e*; boardroom activities associated with, 56–58; described, 43–44; GAAP governing structure/format of, 44, 90; revenue/expense summary on, 44–48, 45*e*; statement of cash flows, 54–55*e*. *See also* Accounting basics; EPFH (E. Polley Francis Hospital)

Financial worthiness, 124

Financing: boardroom activities associated with, 108–109; capital structure ratios and, 71–72, 98–100; creditworthiness and, 100–103; equity and debt sources of, 98; long-term debt, 52–53, 103, 105–108

Financing activities, 55

FitchRatings, 101

Fixed assets (or PPE), 51

The frog in water syndrome, 77

Full financial disclosure, 35

G

GAAP (generally accepted accounting principles): accounting period requirement of, 34; accounting value deter-

mined by, 36; annual audit using, 16; described, 32; financial statements compiled following, 44, 90; unqualified audit opinion and, 132–133*e*

GAAS (generally accepted audit standards), 131

Gapenski, L., 155

GASB (Government Accounting Standards Board), 32

Getting to Great: Principles of Health Care Organization Governance (Pointer and Orlikoff), 154

Governance. *See* Health care organization board governance

"Ground zero" accounting equation, 36

Group-model HMO, 28

H

Health care expenditures: the big picture on, 20–23*e*; distribution for services, 23*e*

Health Care Financing Administration, 27

The Health Care Industry: A Primer for Board Members (Pointer and Williams), 19, 154

Health care organization board governance: dimensions of, 2*e*; "enablers" of, 9–10; resources on, 154–156; specific work of, 8–9*e*; strategic planning as element of, 86–87

Health care organization board policy, 7*e*

Health care organization board roles: decision making, 6, 7*e*; engaging in oversight, 8; financial steward, 142; formulating policies, 6, 7*e*; regarding financial integrity/credibility, 128–129

Health care organization boards: additional tasks of, 5; boardroom tasks of, 10; budgeting involvement by, 94; checklist for, 149–153; "code of conduct" of, 137–138; diversity of, 1; fiduciary duty of loyalty of, 3; financial calendar, 143, 144*e*–146*e*, 147; financial integrity/credibility role of, 128–129; financial performance oversight process by, 77*e*, 78; governance work of, 2*e*, 8–9*e*; helpful resources for, 154–156; obligations of, 2; parting admonitions for, 141–148; responsibilities of, 3–4, 142–143, 147–148; roles of, 6, 8, 10. *See also* Boardroom activities

Health care personnel, 22*e*

Health insurance: described, 23–24; HMO (health maintenance organizations), 25, 28–29; national statistics on, 21*e*; social insurance (Medicare), 24, 26–27; three types of, 24; VHI (voluntary health insurance), 24–26; welfare insurance (Medicaid), 24, 28

Health Insurance Coverage (Bureau of the Census, 2000), 20

Health Insurance Coverage and the Uninsured (Health Insurance Institute of America), 20

Health, United States—2002 (National Center for Health Statistics), 20

Healthcare Finance: An Introduction to Accounting and Financial Management (Gapenski), 155

HFMA (Healthcare Financial Management Association), 32

HFMA Principles and Practice Board, 32

Historical capital investment approach, 113–114

HMO (health maintenance organizations): overview of, 25, 28–29; revenue from operations for, 46

Horizontal financial analysis, 62, 64*e*

Hospitals: HMOs (health maintenance organizations) and, 29; national statistics on, 21*e*–22*e*

I

Income statement, 46

Infrastructure of governance, 10

Insurance. *See* Health insurance

Interest expenses, 47

Interests (coupon) rate, 107

Internal controls, 136

Inventories, 50

Investing activities, 55

Investment banker, 105

Issuing authority, 105

K

Kaufman, K., 155

Key goals: defining, 84; of EPFH (E. Polley Francis Hospital), 85*e*; relation to vision, 83*e*

King, M. L., Jr., 142

Kroc, R., 77

L

Legal counsel, 106

Leverage, 99

Liabilities: balance sheet listing, 51–53; current, 51–52; described, 37; long-term debt, 52–53, 103, 105–108

Liquidity ratios, 66–68

LLCs (limited liability companies), 33

LLPs (limited liability partnerships), 33

Long-term debt (noncurrent liabilities): current portions of, 52; described, 52–53; financing using, 103, 105–108

Long-term investments, 51

M

Mandated capital projects, 115

Market, 105–106

Materiality (accounting), 35

McDonald's, 77

Medicaid: described, 24, 28; revenue from DDRG rate paid by, 46

Medicare, 24, 26–27

Medicare Part A, 26–27

Medicare Part B, 27

Mental/behavioral health statistics, 22*e*

Mimic capital investment approach, 114

Modern Healthcare (magazine), 154

Monetary unit, 34

Moody's Investors Service, 101

Mortgage bond, 106

Municipal bond ("muni" or tax-exempt), 106–107

N

Net accounts receivable, 50
Net cash flow from operations, 55
Net income, 48
Net income from operations, 48
Net nonoperating income, 48
Net present value analysis: calculating, 123e; described, 121–123; structure of, 122e
New initiatives capital projects, 115
Noncurrent assets, 50–51
Nonoperating revenues, 38
Nursing homes statistics, 22e
NYSE (New York Stock Exchange) rules, 136–137

O

Objectivity (accounting), 34
Operating activities, 55
Operating expenses, 47–48
Operating improvement capital projects, 115
Operating margin, 69–70
Operating revenues, 38
Operating statistics, 73–74e
Organizational ends responsibility, 3–4
Orlikoff, J., 154
Owners equity: calculating, 53; debt-to-equity ratio, 71; described, 37; as financing source, 98; return on, 70–71

P

Payback analysis, 120–121e
Payroll accurals, 52
PCs (professional corporations), 33
Physician national statistics, 22e
Placement, 107
Planning: boardroom activities associated with, 95–96; budgeting, 93–94; financial, 87–93; vision and strategic, 82–85e, 86e–87, 124
Planning cycle, 82e
Pointer, D., 19, 154
Political capital investment approach, 114
Popularity capital investment approach, 113

PPE (property, plant, and equipment), 51
Prepaid items, 50
Principles and Practice Board (HFMA), 32
Profitability ratios, 68–71
Provision for uncollectables (bad debt), 48
Public Company Accounting Reform and Investor Protection (Sarbanes-Oxley) Act of 2002, 136, 137
Public welfare insurance, 24

Q

Qualified opinion, 132
Quality of care responsibility, 4

R

Ratio analysis: activity ratios, 72–73; calculating, 65; capital structure ratios, 71–72, 98–100; four types of, 65; liquidity, 66–68; operating statistics used in, 73–74e; profitability, 68–71; trends in using, 74–76, 75e
RBRVS (resource-based relative value scale), 27
Reserve fund, 108
Retirement schedule, 108
Return on equity, 70–71
Revenue budget component, 93–94
Revenues: boardroom activities regarding, 57; days revenue in accounts receivable ratio, 67–68; EPFH revenue/expense summary, 45e, 60e; financial statement summary of, 44–47; operating and nonoperating, 38
Risk: capital project, 116e–117; due to debt, 99
The Role of the Board of Directors in Enron's Collapse (2002), 128

S

Sarbanes-Oxley Act (2002), 136, 137
Securities and Exchange Commission (SEC), 103
Self-funded plans, 25
Social insurance (Medicare), 24, 26–27
Social Security Act (Title 18), 26